Laughing Hearts

Laughing Hearts

my joy-filled heart transplant journey

Linda Savolaine(n) LeVier

Book and Brand Publishing
San Diego, CA

Dedication

To my son, Craig, and daughter, Kristin, who suffered more than I did during the darkest days yet kept the atmosphere around me upbeat throughout my medical journey.

This book is my thank-you to all past and future organ donors who sign up on the Organ Donor Registry, not knowing whether they will be chosen to save a person's life. I feel deep gratitude for my donor and her family for giving me a chance to continue my life at a time when my donor's life was unable to be saved.

The main thing
in one's own private world
is to try to laugh
as much as you cry.

—Maya Angelou

Contents

Foreword

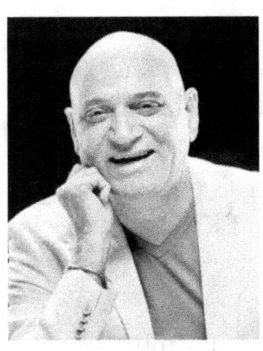

Linda's book on her journey through a heart transplant is a great example of how anyone can "seriously laugh" their way through any challenge thrown by life. While going through the toughest patch, Linda resorted to the best medicine of all times—laughter—and emerged a winner!

I am very touched, moved, and inspired by her book. As a physician, I know that fifty percent of all diseases are organic as there is some incidental cause for sickness, but the other fifty percent is the mental reaction to that disease, especially when it is life threatening or chronic. Therefore, it is very important to keep your mind positive when you go through any difficult situation in life. Laughter Yoga helped Linda keep her spirits high while going through all her heart trouble.

Her narrative of personal experiences is thought provoking and will help to change your perspective through laughter so that you can live a better life. But remember, it is not just about knowing laughter or doing it; it is about living it. Therefore, the best way to get the maximum benefits of laughter is to teach others to be happy. It is essential to bring happiness to others in order to find yourself happy. Well, Linda is doing a great job of that! She has not only laughed herself, but has motivated and helped many others. Her book will be a great inspiration for people in years to come.

I thank Linda for her relentless effort in bringing more laughter into the lives of people, and wish her all the best of health, happiness, and peace.

Always keep laughing and smiling—it takes you a long way in life ... ha ha ha!

Love and laughter,

Dr. Madan Kataria, Founder, Laughter Yoga International

Acknowledgments

I must first acknowledge my strongest cheerleaders, who insisted I had a worthwhile story to tell. Christopher Barry, my nephew, and Edward Savolaine, MD, my cousin, encouraged and pushed me when I hit roadblocks and pleaded with me not to give up.

Sarito Sun, my first laughter leader, set me on a path I could not have imagined when I was in my forties. She and Gaga and Khevin Barnes introduced me to intentional laughing, the least expensive and most beneficial integrative medicine, which I use regularly.

Sarito introduced me to Chiwah Carol Slater when I mentioned that I wanted to write a book about laughter and the immense part it played during my heart transplant journey.

Chiwah displayed compassion and patience as I wrote, hesitated, and bounded forward in an uneven pace for five years. My main excuses involved my good health and the increasing happiness and courage that allowed me to participate in activities I had not attempted earlier in my life. Focusing on my medical roller coaster ride and concentrating on a writing assignment did not stay at the top of my priorities list.

JoAnn Morse and Joni Doyle, neighbors who became dear friends, were the first people I allowed to read the opening chapters as they unfolded. They encouraged me to write the way I talk. They enjoyed my humorous and uplifting take on my serious condition. Most of all, they kept nudging me to keep writing.

My daughter, Kristin, was concerned that my lighthearted writing style might minimize the seriousness of my condition. She encouraged me to help readers feel the anxiety that kept her and her brother from revealing to me negative information they received. Heart-to-heart talks after my hospital stays brought out the true picture of the stress family members often experience when a relative is seriously ill.

The amazing, in-depth notes taken by my son, Craig, when I was in the hospital in 2004 gave me details he recorded to keep his sister informed. As my stay in the hospital lengthened, Craig added the non-medical stories that offered a more complete view of the personal interactions with my family, friends, and medical staff.

Diane Graber stepped in as my family liaison during my transplant surgery. She offered to be with me, realizing that neither my son nor daughter would be able to get to the hospital quickly. The hospital staff gave her pertinent information she passed on to Kristin, who then called Craig.

While Diane kept in touch with my family, she also kept notes to share with me. After my surgery, she presented me with a folder containing her beautifully written account of my heart transplant surgery. She was an over-the-top family liaison who was greatly appreciated.

As publishing my book was becoming a reality, several neighbors helped with proofreading. I appreciate their looking for typos and odd sentence structure, and for their thoughtful general comments. Jane Allen took on the lion's share of this task.

Friends from my Laughter Yoga community told me to share my pre-printed book with Dr. Madan Kataria, the founder of Laughter Yoga. To me, he is a superstar. After I became a Laughter Yoga teacher I sent him notices and stories that showed I'd been utilizing what he'd taught me.

I was overjoyed to receive his warm response to my request that he write the foreword to this book.

My last acknowledgment goes to a free opportunity to laugh with people from anywhere in the world during a ten-to-twenty-minute session. You may just listen. You don't need to give your name. There are several sessions a day, every day of the year. In the Search space of your computer, put Laughter Yoga on the Phone. The site will give you information for how to join others in getting a dose of healthy laughing.

Motorcycle Heart Surgery

A mechanic was removing a cylinder head from the motor of a Harley, when he spotted a world-famous heart surgeon in his shop. The heart surgeon was waiting for the service manager to come take a look at his bike.

The mechanic shouted across the garage, "Hey Doc can I ask you a question?" The famous surgeon, a bit surprised, walked over to the mechanic working on the motorcycle.

The mechanic straightened up, wiped his hands on a rag and asked, "So Doc, look at this engine. I also can open it up, take valves out, fix 'em, put in new parts and when I finish this will work just like a new one. So how come I get a pittance and you get the really big money, when you and I are doing basically the same work?"

The surgeon paused, smiled and leaned over, and whispered to the mechanic, "Try doing it while it's running."

posted June 7, 2016 by Adam Pick at http://www.heart-valve-surgery.com/heart-surgery-blog/2007/09/14/heart-valve-humor-a-cardiac-surgeon-and-a-car-mechanic/

Introduction

Laughing Hearts ... I've had two.

My birth heart laughed easily and often, starting with peek-a-boo and the silly noises coming from those huge bodies that zoomed into my line of sight when I was a baby. I think of my heart laughing when unexpected funny twists occurred, as in a mix-up of words or plans. My heart likes sweet, innocent, and joyful humor.

It's my mind that sets off the laughing when I hear a clever joke or see a comedy sketch. The mind is more likely than the heart to laugh at negative humor, as in watching someone crash into a tree while on a tire swing. Yes, I have had my share of laughing *at* someone's pain or predicament.

I get a better, longer-lasting feeling when I am laughing *with* someone over a slip of the tongue or an unexpected misstep that strikes us both as funny. I love it when my sister starts to laugh at something and can't stop long enough to tell me what set her off. Then I can't help but join in. Whatever started Marilyn laughing never measured up to the fun we had laughing about laughing.

As I got older, there seemed to be less lighthearted opportunities for laughing. I laughed when I was nervous or felt powerless and resorted to sarcastic quips. Thank goodness my own children and my students provided a constant supply of upbeat humorous material!

When I moved to the San Diego area in 1998, after my children were grown, I told friends I was hoping to have a future with more laughing, singing, and dancing. By attending activities at the Carlsbad Senior Center, I got to enjoy all three wishes within two weeks.

Early in the medical journey that began in 2004, one of my doctors said, "You need lots of laughing." I took his words as seriously as if he'd written them on a prescription pad.

I was lucky enough to have doctors and nurses who picked up on my upbeat sense of humor. During my nine weeks in the ICU they joined me in taking every possible opportunity to see humor within the darkness.

I was surprised when laughing opportunities sprang up unexpectedly during the three-month Healing Hearts rehabilitation program I attended after my bypass surgery. I was with people who were very sick and yet found themselves laughing together at off-hand remarks.

I joined the local chapter of a heart disease support group called WomenHeart. I didn't think humor would be a part of the self-help sessions. I'm delighted to report that I was wrong!

I attended other groups that centered around special interests of mine. As the years passed, I realized I had allowed myself to be socially isolated for most of my adult life. I'd interacted with neighbors and other teachers, but had not formed close friendships.

My biggest takeaway after reviewing my life was realizing that my spouse, children, and closest friends should not be expected to meet all my physical and emotional needs. I got insight, compassion, and a lighthearted take on my own stresses, fears, passions, and weaknesses when I heard other people share stories of dealing with their own challenges.

Connecting with Laughter Meditation and Laughter Yoga literally changed my life. One of my supreme life highlights was meeting Dr. Kataria when he came from India to conduct a Laughter Yoga Teacher Training Seminar in Chicago in 2010. I finally understood that it was laughter I was seeking, not humor. He gave me permission to enjoy playfulness whenever my life became unbalanced with too much seriousness.

I looked for laughing opportunities.

I realized that heading to a Laughter Yoga session when I was in pain, physically or emotionally, was far better medicine than taking antidepressants or pain killers. I knew I had been given the best prescription for relief, one that had no nasty side effects.

Now I laugh to achieve a natural high.

My second heart, my transplanted one, has taken full advantage of the act of laughing whenever I've just wanted to feel good. The humor comes after the laughing, as the playfulness sets in.

Don't get me wrong. I will not stop seeing my doctors or taking the heavy-duty medicines I need to regulate my medical conditions. I do believe, however, that there is a real mind/body connection. I think my outlook and the attitudes of my son, my daughter, and most of my medical team played a significant role in making my heart transplant journey truly joy-filled.

The story of my medical journey includes serious details, sweet memories, and spiritual experiences. The majority of my stories make me smile and laugh out loud as I think of the humor and uplifting support from my family and an ever-increasing number of friends. I am truly grateful for the technical, personal, and humorous talents of my medical teams from two hospitals.

As I looked back at that journey, I decided I'd been writing about the contrast between who I was growing up and who I became when I faced my medical challenge. As I evolved into the person I am now, I began to pull strength from my Finnish ancestry and my authentic last name, Savolainen, even though I'd grown up with the non-Finnish-sounding name of Savolaine.

If you find the medical detail too much to endure, feel free to skim the parts that don't interest you. The real gift I intend for you is wrapped in the stories about my experiences and, especially, the wonderfully supportive and caring people who saw me through it all.

I would enjoy hearing from you if you would like to share a reaction to one of my stories. Some people are resigned to letting aging take its course. I want to be with others, face to face and via computer, who choose to associate with people who also have a laughing heart.

LaughingHearts4us@icloud.com

Linda Savolainen LeVier

1

An Innocent Request

Sometimes life is a roller coaster. You can't see the bumpy track, the scary climbs to new heights, or the wild downslopes ahead. You just hang on for dear life.

I grew up a people pleaser, afraid of my own shadow. Too filled with self-doubt to defend my beliefs, I found myself caught between the people I loved when they disagreed with each other. My husband said I sat on the fence so often I must have splinters in my rear.

We raised our family in Glendora, a warm and friendly city in northeast Los Angeles County. While I had good connections with my neighbors, other teachers, and the parents of my children's friends, I developed few strong personal ties. I felt controlled and socially stifled.

It was only as I grew older that I began to open up, to say "yes" to new experiences and people.

Once our children had graduated college and joined the workforce, I felt a need to nurture myself. I had plenty of photos, scrapbooks, and souvenirs to show a past filled with good memories. Yet the atmosphere in our home was nose to the grindstone, look busy even if you're wasting time. There was little joy or playfulness.

I had no idea how many years I had left to live. I just knew I had to have more laughing, singing, and dancing.

The biggest shift in my foundation came in 1998, after my divorce, when I decided to move to San Diego County, where my son lived. I was fifty-eight years old when I moved to Carlsbad, where I lived alone in a small condo complete with ocean view. I felt as if I had died and gone to heaven.

Although I had no trouble amusing myself with reading, music, TV, and other solo activities in this beautiful setting, I knew I was going to need new people and activities to get me out of my home. I was on the

1

young side for going to a senior center. But where else could I meet people during the day?

That first week, I sang with a chorus. I laughed my heart out in an improvisational theater class. At the local farmers' market I bought long-stemmed sunflowers and arranged them in a tall wastebasket I set out on my living room floor.

The second week, I watched seniors much older than I holding their own on the dance floor long after I'd nearly dropped from exhaustion.

My first two years I spent getting to know the area, volunteering at a local school and reentering the world of dating. The dating bolstered my self-esteem, but I was not ready to commit to any one person.

The birth of my first grandchild, Grace, opened up a new place in my heart. I shared the babysitting with my daughter-in-law's family. I saw my son, Craig, take easily to the role of totally committed, loving, involved father. Less than two years later a second little girl, Tori, entered their family. Her full head of dark hair standing straight up over her charming face delighted us. Before my daughter-in-law went back to work, we enjoyed talking about her childhood and other topics.

The baby stayed with the other grandparents while big sister and I went out on adventures during our five days together each week. We enjoyed picnic lunches before I went to a gym class. She met new friends in the gym's playroom. We spent hours at the library, the Wild Animal Park, a pet store, a gym for toddlers, and the mall. We enjoyed playing drums (empty yogurt containers), reading lots of books, and doing art projects.

I will always cherish my close ties with my son's family as they balanced work and parenting. My granddaughters were in good hands, with a large and loving extended family.

Then came the news that my daughter, Kristin, who lived in Michigan, was pregnant! I was invited to join the parents-to-be for the birth, and to stay until my daughter returned to work.

My heart overflowed with love. Soon after learning that I was about to gain a third grandchild, I had a vision—my first one. I had just gotten out of bed for a middle-of-the-night trek to the bathroom when I was surprised, not with a vision, but with an almost-visual message.

I think I said out loud, "Oh! I'm going to have a grandson. That's nice."

The next morning, I remembered the strange event and decided to write the gender of the new baby on a piece of paper and tuck it away. I chose to not say anything about it until after the birth.

It was May of 2003 when I drove myself to Michigan. Before I left, I visited my primary care physician, Dr. Hauser. Responding to the news of the potentially harmful side effects of long-term use of estrogen replacement, we discontinued my hormone therapy.

"I am woman. Hear me roar!" became my mantra.

The trip plans evolved into the added fun of taking a college friend with me to Santa Fe, New Mexico, to stay with another college friend. In Santa Fe I also visited a friend I'd met during an Elderhostel week. The drive, the tourist fun, the talking and laughing were a great beginning for this adventure.

Of course my uppermost thought was, "Baby, don't come early."

I drove the rest of the way alone. I had never done a long drive alone. I truly enjoyed the drive, the motel nights, the audio books, and the good feeling of having accepted the challenge of the drive. Better yet, the baby did not come early. In fact, I enjoyed several days with my daughter while she was on maternity leave and the baby was content with life in the womb.

All birth experiences are unique. I was surprised to learn that I would be with my daughter for the labor and the birth, along with the medical staff and Brian, my son-in-law. A special bonus for me was seeing Brian serve as a tender and loving labor coach.

It was a long labor. When at last the baby came, the doctor said, "It's a boy." Immediately, both my daughter and I called out, "I knew it!"

A few days later, my son-in-law showed me the envelope with the paper they had tucked away without ever looking at it. On the paper the nurse had written "BOY" after an ultrasound. I told them about my piece of paper, with "I'm going to have a grandson" written on it!

The next three months were packed with local fun, a trip to Ohio for a wedding, and a visit from my son and his family. I was overjoyed as I watched my granddaughters welcome their new cousin, Aengus. Our last big adventure involved a road trip to Wyoming.

My sister, Marilyn, arrived at the end of my visit in the Midwest to see her new nephew and accompany me on the drive back to California. Before she arrived I was beginning to feel more tired than usual. Though I trudged daily up and down the stairs of my daughter's multi-storied home with the baby in my arms, I was off my exercise routine and missed my trainer. (I have no self-discipline.) I had never been an athlete, but I'd always been careful about weight gain and maintaining good health.

We made the return drive to California in August. I went back to working with my trainer, but I wasn't getting stronger. It felt as if my knees and ankles were breaking down. My energy was low, and I was becoming depressed. My doctor prescribed physical therapy. That helped my aches, but did nothing for my energy level or my emotions.

In January, I added yoga and a second trainer. I grew a little stronger, but my energy level was still low. Achy and gaining weight, I began to feel like a broken woman. I don't believe I shared that thought with my doctor.

My depression continued, so I went to see Dr. Hauser again in February. Years later, I sent for doctors' notes and hospital records to refer to as I wrote this book. I found it interesting that she'd noted on that visit that I lacked my typical enthusiasm, especially given that I was so happy about having witnessed the birth of my daughter's first child.

Making sure I understood the risks, she reinstated the hormone replacement therapy.

Just twelve days later, on March 10th, 2004, I returned for my yearly physical. The hormone therapy must have helped, because my mood had lifted and my knees and ankles felt better. "I'm back!" I told her. No depression, no aches. Nothing suspicious showed up during the in-office exam.

As my doctor stood with her hand on the doorknob, ready to leave the examining room, I suddenly blurted, "Could I have a treadmill test?"

"What?"

I repeated my question. "Could I have one of those treadmill tests?"

Dr. Hauser did a double take. "A stress test? Why? You are one of my healthiest patients."

I became flustered, unable to remember why I had planned to request this test. Many months later, my daughter-in-law reminded me about an article I had read in a women's magazine. There was a list of medical tests and recommendations for the age at which women should have each test. There it was: "Women in their sixties should have a treadmill stress test." I'd thought it would be a good idea to get some guidance as to what physical activities would be best for me.

My doctor asked me questions about my family history. My father had died at age fifty. It was his heart that had given out, after eight years of health problems that began during World War II when he was a Navy Seabee on the Pacific Front.

I also told her about my sister, who had died at the age of forty. Again, it was her heart that gave out, after a long battle with mostly undiagnosed medical issues. My father's and sister's health histories were apparently not related.

My doctor's next question: "Have you ever had any symptoms of heart problems?"

"Well," I replied, "several years ago I began to have short phases of numbness in my left arm." I had told my doctors, including her, about the numbness, and they had said that a slightly pinched nerve was probably the cause, since the symptom faded as soon as there was any distraction or stress release.

Even though I wasn't concerned about my heart, and my doctor didn't seem to be, either, the information I gave led her to schedule a stress test for me on March 29th.

2

They Won't Let Me Go Home

When the big day came, I sat calmly in the waiting room. I learned that I would have to wait a while, as the staff had not noticed that I was to have a stress test with an EKG,[1] and there was only one room with the proper equipment.

"No problem," I said. "I have a book to read."

Mine was the last appointment of the day. I put on the gown. Electrodes were stuck onto various parts of my body. Then I sat and waited … and waited … while the technician looked at the screen. I couldn't see what had caught his attention. At one point I asked, "Aren't I supposed to get on the treadmill?"

Finally, he told me to go over to the equipment. We started with a slow walk. After about a minute he asked me, "Are you all right?"

"Yes."

Nevertheless, he told me to get off and sit down. A second person came in to look at the monitor, and then a third person. It seemed that I sat a long time before the technician instructed me to get back on the treadmill.

Again, the plodding commenced. This second time on the treadmill seemed even shorter than the first, though hospital records show that I completed a total of six minutes, forty-five seconds.

I was told to get off the treadmill and put on my street clothes.

None of this weird scenario made me nervous. Curious? Yes. Nervous? No.

I was putting on my street clothes when the nurse came in and asked me, "Would you mind if I bring a doctor in to see you?"

---

[1] According to WebMD.com, an electrocardiogram (EKG or ECG) is a test that checks for problems with the electrical activity of your heart, as in rapid or irregular heartbeats (palpitations), and determines whether the walls of the heart chamber are too thick.

My funny, twisted mind thought, Is he good looking?

In came Dr. Rubenson, a cardiologist. His expression was pleasant, but his tone was serious when he said, "We would like to have you spend the night."

"Oh, I can't," I replied. "I have to babysit tomorrow."

Then, reconsidering, I asked whether I could call my son, Craig. "I don't think I can babysit tomorrow," I told him. "Will that be okay?"

"No problem. We'll work something out. What's going on?" Craig said later that I'd sounded a bit choked up, possibly teary.

"I'm in the hospital. They won't let me go home. They want to do another test that will give information beyond what the treadmill test showed."

The conversation with my primary care physician had led her to request a stress test with an EKG. I had considered the test no more out of the ordinary than a routine mammogram or PAP test.

Years later, I learned from the hospital records that the notes before the treadmill test showed no red flags:

> **Hospital Records, March 29, 2004**
> Heart rate, 72; blood pressure 140/80; the mean venous pressure normal for a healthy-appearing youthful female in no acute distress. The current pre-treadmill EKG is normal.

The post-treadmill notes, especially item number three, showed a totally different picture. In summary:

> ASSESSMENT:
> 1. Hypertension under borderline control
> 2. A 13-year history of atypical arm discomfort
> 3. Significantly abnormal stress test with wall motion abnormalities and ST segment depression
> 4. History of migraine-like headaches
> 5. Mild hypercholesterolemia with LDL of 123

I was told I should have an angiogram[1] the next day to confirm the diagnosis, at which time I would hear the plan for appropriate therapy.

---

[1] An angiogram, or cardiac catheterization, is an X-ray of the coronary arteries that is taken after injecting dye through a catheter.

After learning about the procedure, the risks, and the alternatives, I gave my consent to stay in the hospital overnight. I don't think I heard any of the technical medical terms, but the tone was serious enough for me to agree to the follow-up test.

* * *

I don't recall being taken to a hospital room. I vaguely remember reading the book I happened to have with me. I do not remember having dinner, though I suppose I did. Then again, maybe I didn't, since I was going to have further testing the next day.

I do recall that Liz, a soft-spoken woman, came to my room and offered to do a relaxation technique called Healing Touch. While I was not familiar with that treatment, I knew a little about Reiki, a relaxation method a good friend of mine had experienced. I was quick to accept her offer.

I think I was on my stomach the whole time. She leaned over me and moved her hands above my body, up and down the full length. We didn't converse. I remember her leaving my room. That was it. Out like a light.

I have learned more about Healing Touch since my first experience, and highly recommend the treatment to others.

* * *

The angiogram was performed at Scripps Green Hospital in La Jolla.

After receiving a call at work from Dr. Curtis, another cardiologist, Craig began to take detailed notes to share with Kristin. Little did he realize he would be keeping a written record of an extensive medical adventure. I will let Craig's notes tell some of the story, in this format:

Craig's Notes

TUESDAY, MARCH 30

Dr. Curtis called me at work to detail the findings of the angiogram. To everyone's surprise, he found the narrowing and blocking of the arteries severe enough to recommend bypass surgery.

There. Welcome to my roller coaster. Hang tight to your seat! You are in for a ride.

> Mom accepted the recommendation, and bypass[1] surgery was scheduled for tomorrow morning (March 31st).
>
> Basically, Mom's heart is not getting enough blood.
>
> • Left anterior descending artery - 90% narrowing
>
> • Left circumflex artery - 80 % narrowing
>
> • Right coronary artery - 100% blocked; has had a silent heart attack.
>
> The damage started long ago and has probably been getting progressively worse over the years.
>
> Dr. Housman, cardiac surgeon, will perform the surgery, which can take from two and a half to four hours.

I had no clue I'd had a silent heart attack. No wonder I was always feeling so tired!

* * *

Craig was with me after the angiogram, from 12:30 to 6:30pm. He remembers the afternoon as uneventful. His notes indicate that we passed the time talking and making a few phone calls.

I received a call from my daughter after Craig left. He had left her a message telling her she didn't need to call me, adding, "Mom doesn't want anyone to be concerned."

Recently, my daughter told me, "The night before your bypass surgery, I was at a movie with a friend. Since my son was less than a year old, this was probably the first movie I had seen in over a year. I got a message when I came home that you were going to have a 'simple bypass operation' that was expected to go smoothly the next day. Craig said I didn't need to call you, that you didn't want to bother or worry anyone, and that you didn't want us to tell people about the surgery. Even though it was late when I got the message, I called you anyway."

Kristin added, "You told me how good your prognosis was because of your good health. I believed you, but I couldn't believe you didn't want me to call you. I was surprised that you did not seem at all concerned."

[1] During coronary artery bypass graft surgery (also called CABG, or "cabbage"), a blood vessel is removed or redirected from one area of the body and placed around the area or areas of narrowing in order to "bypass" the blockages and restore blood flow to the heart muscle.

I don't remember any of this. I was reminded much later of Kristin's call. No one, especially me, seemed to have any concern about what was to take place the next morning.

3

Get the Pee Queen

The message that I would need bypass surgery was delivered in a calm manner. While serious, bypass surgery was nothing unusual. The fact that my general health was good and my heart was strong meant there was only a one- to two-percent chance of incurring complications.

Before bed I had an enjoyable conversation with the woman who again offered her gift of Healing Touch. I awoke rested, and received a pleasant call from my son before I left for the bypass surgery.

I do not remember signing permission papers for bypass surgery. Certainly fear would have reared its ugly face at that time. Yet I have no recollection of being afraid.

Over the years I have realized that I have a high pain threshold, meaning that I tolerate pain rather well. On the other hand, I have a very low fear threshold. If I think I will be in pain, I start feeling pain, emotionally or physically, before the painful event occurs. If I am told that I will have a dental procedure in a week or two, I will experience fear and pain in my gums before the event. Then I will experience little or no pain during the actual dental work.

That is why I have repeatedly asked my son, "Was I freaking out?"

"No," is the response I always get.

Why was I not freaking out? If nothing else, my need for bypass surgery should have taken my mind back to the deaths of my father and sister. Both of them had suffered complex medical conditions that ended with their hearts giving out.

✶ ✶ ✶

The doctors told Craig that my heart was quite healthy, that it was just the arteries that were no good. Particularly because of my generally good health, they said, the risk of this procedure was very low.

After the surgery patients could expect to remain in the hospital for about five days, the first day or two of which would be in the ICU. Physical therapy would begin in the hospital and continue at home. Cardiac rehabilitation was recommended. The majority of the recovery usually happened in three to four weeks, with gradually increasing activity. Heavy lifting should be avoided for two months.

* * *

My son called me at 5:30 the next morning to wish me well with the bypass surgery. He noted that I sounded great and that I told him I had slept well all night, probably thanks to the gift of Healing Touch the night before.

My only pre-surgery memory begins with watching a nurse try to insert my urinary catheter. I heard some murmuring, and then a second nurse arrived to help. Upon the arrival of a third nurse, I heard, "Get the Pee Queen." A few minutes later the "Pee Queen," a nurse with a unique gift for inserting catheters, arrived. The catheter was smoothly inserted, and I was soon rolling down the hall to the operating room with a smile on my face.

* * *

The surgery began around 8:00. Expecting it to take two and a half to four hours, Craig settled down in the waiting room.

An attending nurse called him at 11:45 and said the expected four grafts (bypasses) were completed and everything was going well. They were "closing" now, and the doctor would be out to talk with him in thirty to forty minutes.

At 12:30pm, not long after Craig had called Kristin to pass on the good news, Craig got another call from the OR with the message that they needed to harvest another vein because one of the grafts "didn't take." They told him they expected to be done in thirty minutes.

Craig grew nervous when two hours passed with no further information. As his waiting time grew longer, what was he thinking? Not expecting anything unusual to happen, he waited alone. My son is a calm, levelheaded guy. I can't speak for what he was feeling inside.

Craig's Notes, based on info from Dr. Housman

WEDNESDAY, MARCH 31

As they were closing (at about the time I got the call that everything was fine), the EKG and other diag-

---

> nostics showed that two of the grafted veins had collapsed. This can happen for a number of reasons, including the body's own reaction to the change, a response to the anesthesia, etc. Once this happens, however, they do not trust those grafted veins, so they perform another graft while keeping the first ones in place.

It was 2:40 in the afternoon when Dr. Housman called to tell Craig that I was fine.

> Ultimately, there were five bypasses—three at one site and one at each of two other sites. Things look stable now, but they have her on a balloon pump[1] to give her heart a rest. They want her to rest overnight, so she will be unconscious until tomorrow.
>
> The doctor said I could wait an hour or so for them to finish up and get her back to the ICU. Then I could go up to see her.

Craig left after seeing me, at about 4:00pm.

At 7:30 that evening Craig got a call from Dr. Rubenson during which he learned that I was heading to the cath lab, with its diagnostic imaging equipment, to see why I was taking so long to recover from the bypass surgery.

> Dr. Rubenson started by saying that Mom was fine. However, he was concerned that one graft might not have taken. He said she had not gotten any worse since the surgery, but had not gotten better as quickly as they had hoped.
>
> He said that after a conversation with Dr. Housman, the surgeon, they had decided to see what was flowing and what was not. They might not find anything, but would feel better if they checked. If they found a block, they could possibly clear it with a balloon at that time. They would call again when they knew more.
>
> Working together, they found that nearly all the grafts and native vessels were clotted. Dr. Teirstein was summoned to insert stents. During a call at 10:15pm Dr. Housman told me, "The grafts look much better now. We put in seven stents to open the passage-ways."

[1] A balloon pump is a mechanical device that increases coronary blood flow and oxygen supply.

> Because of all of this, she will not be awake in the morning. I can go in at my leisure.

* * *

Seven stents![1] Thank goodness I'd been allowed to have the treadmill test. Given that I had an HMO insurance policy, I don't think my request would have been granted had it not been for the deaths of my father and sister ... and the fact that I had experienced numbness in my left arm.

It was a bittersweet fact that the deaths of my sister Jean and my daddy, who died when I was ten, played a part in saving my life.

---

[1] Stents are small expandable tubes used to treat narrowed or weakened arteries in the body. Stent procedures usually involve balloon angioplasty. They use a long, thin tube called a catheter that has a small balloon on its tip. They inflate the balloon at the blockage site in the artery to flatten or compress the plaque against the artery wall.

4

Medically Induced Coma

Craig's Notes

THURSDAY, APRIL 1

5:20am: I called the ICU and spoke to Michelle, Mom's attending night shift nurse. She said, "Your mother is doing okay, but she is on a lot of medication." She also detailed last night's events that led to inserting seven stents. "Your mother will probably be on medication and knocked out all day to let her heart and body rest. As soon as the ventilator tube comes out of her throat, she will be able to wake up."

Michelle told me that Mom "did wake up briefly, and she acknowledged the nurse prior to going downstairs to the cath lab yesterday evening, so she is definitely fine 'up there'" (mentally).

She has fourteen drips (IV medications) going right now. Best thing is to rest her heart. They know how well things are going by the IV in her neck, and can tell how each part of the heart is doing.

That was the day Craig met Dr. Curtis, cardiologist, for the first time. He learned that the heart was still healthy, particularly the lower portion with the three bypasses.

The doctors had said that after recovery I would probably be better than before, because of the increased blood flow to the heart. But Craig had also heard that X-rays and an echocardiogram[1] might show damage

---

[1] An echo/echocardiogram gives a graphic outline of the heart's movement. Ultrasound technology accurately visualizes the motion of the heart's walls and pumping action under stress. The test may reveal a lack of blood flow that isn't apparent on other heart tests. The test result is called "ejection fraction," expressed as a percentage.

that had occurred between the time of the bypass surgery and the insertion of the stents.

He was pleased to hear that there should be no long-term effects from all the drugs they were giving me to help me rest.

> 8:00pm phone conversation with Michelle, Mom's night nurse: "Still the same with 14 IV drips."
>
> Another doctor called me at 9:30pm. Her vitals are dropping off a bit. They will try to change the situation with medication over the next ten to fifteen minutes. If no improvement, they might take her back to the cath lab to find out what is wrong. I said okay to that.
>
> But they decided against it, as she is improving with the meds and they don't want to introduce any unnecessary risk.
>
> They changed some of the medications, and her numbers are the best ever. They like "index numbers[1] greater than 2," Mom's level when she entered the ICU. Now they are at 2.5, which makes Michelle happy.

Craig wrote a personal note that this was a very long night at their house. It had started to rain, and Tori couldn't sleep.

Michelle told Craig the next morning that I was doing well. The heart had taken over well after she had removed five of the remaining heart drug drips, leaving just four! She added that the index number was 2.7, the best so far, and going in the right direction.

> **Craig's Notes**
>
> FRIDAY, APRIL 2
>
> As for long-term damage, it is still too early to tell. If she continues to improve like she is doing now, they might be able to remove the ventilator tube late this afternoon and she could wake up tonight.
>
> 4:45pm: Dr. Curtis called.
>
> They did another echo today and it looks like things are working. About two-thirds of the heart is contracting and one-third is not. This compares to one-third contracting before.

[1] The term "index numbers" refers to the combination of several individual statistics that are averaged to quantify a patient's overall condition.

> That bodes well for the future. Therefore the sugges-
> tion is to continue on the current path with external
> support, possibly through the weekend.

A doctor told Craig they were not concerned about me dying there; they were just concerned about how impaired I might be when this was all over. Possibilities ranged from a bed-and-chair existence to full recovery. I could have ended up bedridden forever. I can't imagine my daughter and son internalizing that horrifying information.

> It looks like the difficulty came up because all the
> grafts were clotted. This cannot be foreseen before
> surgery. Best index of success is how many drugs
> and external support systems they are able to wean.
>
> 10:00pm – I came in to visit and to meet Michelle.
> She was wonderful! She explained things well and
> was happy to take the time to answer all my ques-
> tions and give her perspective based on past experi-
> ence.
>
> Mom looked good. Her hands were warm. She had
> good color and just looked like she was sleeping,
> much better than a few days ago.
>
> Mom's liver and kidneys are doing great and have
> been doing well all along. Those often do not do well
> in this type of situation, so this is encouraging.

An external pacemaker and a balloon pump were among the support devices monitoring and assisting my heart to beat rhythmically and pump oxygen.

Craig wrote that Michelle had told him she would handpick day and night nurses for us and do her best to convey what she had found to work best over the last few days. He thanked her for this, as well as for her clear communication and wonderful demeanor throughout this ordeal.

Michelle reassured Craig by saying I was doing well and coming around surprisingly quickly. She marked up a diagram of the heart to show him where the bypasses were and where the stents were placed. Overall, she was highly optimistic and admitted that was not something she usually said.

Craig left feeling much better about everything after this visit.

✶ ✶ ✶

The Saturday, April 3rd, notes tell of very slow progress but contain no negative information.

19

In the evening Craig was told that I was tolerating the feeding tube that had been inserted through my nose and down my throat.

On Sunday a nurse told Craig, "Today looks like a good day, but as sick as your mother is, be prepared for a bad day here and there."

Craig's Notes

MONDAY, APRIL 5, one week after the treadmill test

They tried to decrease the balloon pump ratio to 1:3 for an hour. "Your mother basically tolerated it all right," the nurse said, "but the index did drop, as you might expect." Her index had been up as high as 2.6 through the night and dropped to about 2.3 during the trial. All the other labs looked good, so the rest of the systems still seem to be working all right.

12:20pm: I spoke with Dr. Delaria, a cardiac surgeon. "There was no difference from the last echo," he said. "However, your mother has shown enough progress that even without further significant improvement she should be able to take care of herself and keep out of the hospital."

Certain parts of the heart are not working now, but it is not clear whether they will start working after some time, as with a strain to a shoulder muscle. Just need time to tell. Therefore a full recovery is a good wish and still a possibility, but not a given.

There is a wide range of recovery possibilities at this point. Progress has been just right, according to the weekend game plan. She no longer needs a pace-maker (external) because her heart has settled down into a good rhythm.

A doctor said that now was the time to take out the balloon pump and start the slow process of waking me up over the next twenty-four hours. He warned Craig that I would not be rational for thirty-six to forty-eight hours.

The goal now was for me to prove I was okay without the external pump and to get me off the remaining medications. Then it would be time to wake me up and get me moving around, as keeping me sedated for too long could lead to other complications.

She is still on the ventilator. I now understand that the balloon pump helps the heart but is separate from the breathing tube, or ventilator, which breathes for her. She is still sedated, and will be through the rest of the

---

> day and probably the night. They will probably try to wean her off the sedatives tomorrow.

Since the echo had not shown any change, they told Craig I might be limited in my activity later on because of the damage to my heart through all this activity.

Craig's Notes

TUESDAY, APRIL 6

9:00am: Opens eyes occasionally and her pupils act correctly, but no real response. They are using a sedative that can go away quickly.

12:00 noon: The bed is inclined to a sitting position. They have eliminated one of the drugs. She has demonstrated that she can breathe on her own a little bit.

4:30pm: She has definitely been breathing on her own. They have not yet taken out the ventilator, because she has not responded to the verbal commands. She has been responding well to the liquid nourishment.

Craig wrote that he had asked for a possible timetable of events. Bruce, the physician's assistant, had said the tube would probably come out in the next twenty-four hours. Then I would slowly get off the rest of the IV meds and external help.

Bruce had said I should be able to start taking pill medication and eating on my own. They would be watching how I progressed, since my systems had not had to work for a while. He'd predicted I might be in the ICU for perhaps another week.

Physical therapy would be a big next step, because I was "weak as a kitten" after being in bed for a week.

Nurse Leigh Anne had hung a poster in my ICU room. Craig had prepared and printed it, with large photos of each of my three grandchildren. On the bottom were the words "We Love You, Grandma!"

Leigh Anne wanted me to be able to see it easily when my eyes were ready for a beautiful sight. The poster had special meaning and healing benefits for me, and it became a smile producer for all who entered my room.

Craig arrived for a full-day visit on Wednesday.

Craig's Notes

WEDNESDAY, APRIL 7

I saw her open her eyes for the first time, around 11:00am! This happens when the nurse speaks loudly and makes the request for her to open her eyes. Doing so was very labored, however, and she did not respond to "squeeze my hand."

There is no way to know whether she suffered a neurological event when her blood pressure was not what it should have been. If she hasn't awakened by tomorrow, they will do some tests.

Dr. Rubenson says he never expected so many complications. He said the alternative of doing nothing was not a good option either, since with the clogging she had, a heart attack would have gotten her quickly. That would have been that.

Each delay increased my family's stress levels.

11:45am: I got the most response from Mom so far. She opened both eyes when I said, "Mom! I'm here! Can you open your eyes for me?" She has done this several more times, and looks ever closer to waking up, but she's not there yet. She has also shown that she can breathe completely on her own in short tests.

They got her off more drugs. Down to one! Still very sleepy.

The critical care doctor told Craig that I was waking up well within a reasonable time frame after coming off the sedative. I guess I was waking up more whenever they moved me, but then I'd go right back to sleep.

Craig's Notes

THURSDAY, APRIL 8

9:30am: I arrive for a full day of visiting. She still seems sleepy but is definitely waking up and has been moving her arms and legs. She is doing so well off the drugs that they plan to pull the pulmonary IV from her neck . . . the big one.

She does look a bit sick to me. Pale complexion. They won't know the results for a few days from a culture that was taken.

Two blood specialists came by. They are trying to

> figure out why her blood was clotting so aggressively during and after surgery.
>
> 1:00pm: Mom is really seeming to wake up more. She is moving both arms and legs, and even opening her eyes on her own occasionally.
>
> One of the critical care physicians says that most indicators are there for her being able to come off the ventilator, but there is still a concern about her strength and drive: strength to take good deep breaths and the drive to do so as the drugs continue to wear off.
>
> He says she breathes fine when she is awake, but sometimes does not breathe as regularly as she ought to when she goes back to sleep. This is due to the lingering drugs.

Right here, Craig made the switch from always writing about me in third person to mostly writing to me directly. I think that's exciting!

> 5:00pm: You are waking up more and more, with short naps in between. You do a good job of squeezing my hands with both of yours, and also wiggling your toes. You respond well by nodding and shaking your head, but I know it is horribly difficult to not be able to speak.

Yes! You see how well my son understands his talkative mother!

> It is difficult for me to see you grimace in pain, but I am relieved to see you responding to the world.
>
> Your biggest smile came when I told you Kristin and baby Aengus were going to come visit you.
>
> 6:00pm: Dr. Rubenson said he is pleased with the progress but we still need to take it slowly.

It's hard to believe, but at this point it had been a full month since my innocent request for a treadmill test.

Craig noted that I seemed frustrated because I couldn't communicate well with the tube in my mouth, and I didn't have enough strength to use hand motions.

Once I could talk, I had to tell Craig about the two dreams I'd had while I was asleep! I don't recall this, but he wrote that I'd also asked about my sister, Marilyn, and that he'd told me that other than being very concerned for me, she was fine.

He wrote that the next thing I said was, "What a day!"

> After going to your house to take care of things like paying property taxes, listening to messages, and watering plants, I returned to the hospital. You were exhausted from a full day of physical and respiratory therapy.

Everyone seemed to think I'd done very well. Craig wrote that they are amazed at my progress, and that Bruce had said that since I seemed to be swallowing so well, there should be no need to put in a feeding tube. Craig also wrote that I seemed to have developed a good appetite, that I handled the gelatin, energy drink, and yogurt well.

> 9:15pm: The night nurse called and told me there were some complications around 8:00pm. She said your heart stopped beating briefly, but that the external pacemaker was activated immediately. You are fine now. They have also put a breathing mask on to make sure you breathe well. Fortunately, they did not have to reintroduce the ventilator tube.

> My wife and I are disappointed that we could not have
> one full happy day.
>
> I do not know whether it was the right decision, but
> I decided not to call Kristin (past midnight her time)
> with this news since they said the event was so brief
> and not damaging. I'll call both the hospital and Kris-
> tin first thing in the morning.
>
> Looking up at the portrait of your mother for some
> time, my wife asked her to help you.

My heart had stopped beating. Get that? And right after Bruce had said I was doing well! My roller coaster car had chugged up the hill, perched at the top, and then ... oh, no! A quick downturn. But just a short one. Thank heaven for that external pacemaker!

But ... why, oh why, couldn't they have enjoyed just one full happy day?

For the bypass surgery, the insertion of the stents, the induced sleep, and my awakening, the story is about my family and my medical team. Complications arose, and minutes turned into hours and days as obstacles were confronted and overcome.

Perhaps you have experienced a state of disbelief while watching someone in a medically induced coma. I cannot imagine what feelings my son endured as medical personnel kept saying, "She needs one more day of rest" again and again. Or "We cannot say for sure what her physical or mental prognosis is." Or "There are signs that she may have a complete re-covery, but we can't be sure." While Kristin was comfortable revealing her private thoughts years later to me and to readers of my book, Craig chose not to share his personal thoughts.

Put yourself in my daughter's place, living more than halfway across the country. She was told not to call me before the bypass surgery because the odds of an easy surgery were in my favor. I didn't want to worry any-one. Then, bit by bit, her brother called with scary news. When she wanted to come to the hospital right away, she was told not to come because there was nothing she could do while I slept.

I'm aware now that she became physically ill due to the stress she felt. While Craig was hearing from the doctors and nurses the range of pos-sibilities for my recovery, Kristin was getting the shorter versions, without the comforting tones or body language that might have helped her feel better. Her painful memories of those days included not being with Craig to help him and not being able to see or touch me. Can you imagine the feelings of helplessness that must have haunted her?

The medical staff may have used the phrases "needed rest" or "a deep sleep," but the scarier thought "coma" was what Kristin could not get out of her head. Craig took note of possible positive outcomes, while Kristin couldn't get past "She may have brain damage," "She may spend the rest of her life in a wheelchair," and "She may never wake up."

Kristin told me, "The experience was truly terrifying. I thought or worried about you every waking minute during that time, even while supposedly working full time and taking care of Aengus. It was a kind of trance-like existence."

My son and my daughter each had a spouse, offspring under the age of five, and a full-time occupation. How were they supposed to function normally at work, be there for their families, and traverse the rocky road with looming potholes as their mother lay there not participating?

As my hospitalization time lengthened, Craig added the tasks of getting my mail, canceling appointments, paying bills, and fielding calls from family members and friends who were beginning to hear about my situation. Since he couldn't find my mailbox key, he had to sweet-talk the mail carrier into giving him my overflowing mail.

Kristin added, "My brother and I talked so often. We had no idea how to feel when we were told again and again that you needed to stay 'asleep' longer. I felt terrible being far away from you, though we agreed that there was nothing I could do if I did come out to San Diego."

When Craig was given estimates of the time required for the surgery and hospital stay, he was not prepared for the induced sleep. Hearing that I would be asleep for most of the day after the surgery was not alarming. But the sleeping day of April 1st was extended to the next day, and then four days more as my heart made distressingly slow progress toward beating on its own.

Kristin said the calls from Craig were agonizing. The first positive sign was on April 7th when I opened my eyes briefly. There were two more days of eye opening and hand squeezing before I was truly awake, alert, and ready to act out my part in the drama.

Throughout the nine days I was asleep, there was concern about what my mental capacity would be when I woke up. As soon as the breathing tube was removed, I started to talk. After one therapy session, I went right back to talking!

I couldn't wait to share the dream I'd had in the deep sleep. While I don't know the significance of the various parts of the dream, I do think there are some odd pieces.

The dream started with a gal-pals' trip to San Francisco with my former teaching partner, Sherry. (She and I had never taken a trip together. Most of our shared time had been spent enthusiastically planning activities and room environment for our kindergarteners. Sherry died a couple of years before this dream. I can't think of any connection we had with San Francisco. In my dream, we were having a good time.)

The second dream was stranger yet. I was on a Native American reservation. I had just given birth. I remember thinking, within the dream, "How nice to have a baby at the same time Kristin and Craig have young children." Immediately, within the dream, I thought, "Are you crazy? You are sixty-three!"

Then I was standing in a meeting room, in front of a tribal council. I was told about a woman on the reservation who was planning to steal my baby. I was quickly reassured by the elders that I would be given help to escape.

In the last scene I remember, I was racing away on a white horse, presumably clutching my baby. My baby's face was not visible at any point in the dream, nor did I refer to my baby by name.

Up to the time of my dream I'd had no personal connection to a reservation, though I had gone to a few Indian pow-wows. I loved the music, the food, and the dancing.

As for horses, I had always been afraid of them. I'd had a chance to ride a horse on a couple of occasions with friends and my family. Each time I'd declined the offer; I had not had the courage to try riding, not even on the tamest horse alongside a group of parents and little kids. Yet in my dream I was riding away, confidently, with my baby in my arms.

Dream interpreters: Welcome to my inner world!

✶ ✶ ✶

As you read the next chapters you will learn about the personality shifts, good and bad, that can take place when a person is gravely ill or intensely stressed. I want to share some of the coping tools I developed along the way. First and foremost, laughter and humor were always helpful.

Most assuredly, the stress does not stop for those emotionally connected to the patient. When should they offer help or sympathy? When should they back away to allow the patient to test her independence? Should they hover? Give space? Be encouraging cheerleaders? Give reminders about the doctor's orders?

I'm thinking of patients in the hospital. Recovery after a hospital stay is an entirely different can of worms. It can be difficult for caretakers, family members, and close friends to witness the personality changes patients may exhibit as they adjust to physical limitations on their road to recovery.

5

First Days Out of Deep Resting State

The morning of April 10th, during Craig's first talk with Cody, the night nurse, he took down the following information: "Your mother asked, early in the morning, to have the breathing mask removed. She said her mother had come to visit her the previous night. She added, 'That's interesting, because my mother died in 1987. But it was a nice visit.'"

To this day, I can still remember seeing Cody bend down toward me and hearing her say, "Thank you for sharing your story with me."

Yes, that was the morning after my daughter-in-law had looked at the portrait of my mother and asked her to help me.

I clearly remember my mother's visit. Was it a dream? Did it happen at the time my heart stopped beating? You can think whatever feels comfortable to you. The visit took place in the house where we lived before I graduated college, not in my mother's last home. I saw her sitting on a comfortable upholstered chair, across from me. We had a casual conversation about nothing in particular. It reminded me of our first minutes together when I'd come home during a college break.

Wouldn't you think my mother would have encouraged me to be strong and beat this medical challenge? She was not the cheerleading, go-get-'em type. When I was in high school and college she was more inclined to say, "You don't have to get all A's." At various stages in my life I'd felt she didn't believe in my ability to do as well as my sisters or cousins. I felt guilty that I sometimes took the easy road, rather than challenging myself.

At other times, I realized she just wanted to protect me. I was fast-talking, wiggly, twitchy, nervous, and sensitive. I had told my doctors that I'd often felt I was like tightly coiled wire.

My mother had experienced terrible losses. Even though she and her father lived into their eighties, my father died at age fifty. My older sister Jean had died at the tender age of forty. I also had a brother who died when he was four, before I was born. Their deaths were unrelated medically. For my remaining sister and me, my mother leaned toward providing an atmosphere with stress reduction rather than enthusiastic encouragement.

> **Craig's Notes**
>
> SATURDAY, APRIL 10
>
> Today was not a good day. Nurse X was horrible.
>
> You told me the day started with her bringing in your breakfast tray and then leaving. You were so weak at this point that you could not begin to feed yourself, much less peel a banana.
>
> When I called in the morning to see how things were going, the nurse told me you were frustrated because you had dropped your banana, so they had aborted any attempts at physical therapy.
>
> You had to wear an oxygen mask all day, and you had no energy.

My version of the incident: I remember a pleasant staff member bringing in my breakfast tray. I looked at the carton of milk, the cereal, the banana, the straw, the dishes and flatware. Now what? How am I going to be able to eat? I can barely handle the heavy remote I use to call a nurse.

I sat there for a long time. Finally, the nurse looked in, and then backed out of my room. I felt helpless, and then angry. After another long time, the nurse looked in again and started to leave.

"Hey!" I yelled. Okay, I admit I was not very polite or respectful. She came back in, and I sputtered, "Have you read my chart?"

So, did I throw the banana or drop it? I don't remember what happened next. Maybe my son arrived and helped me eat.

After all the wonderful doctors and nurses my son had come to know, I started my recovery with the one bad seed who had probably just overslept and gotten up on the wrong side of the bed that morning. The charge nurse assured Craig that Nurse X would not be assigned to me in the future.

✴ ✴ ✴

As if Craig didn't have enough problems, he heard from my nephew in San Francisco that there was a medical problem with my sister, Marilyn. She had planned to come to San Diego to be my main visitor so that Craig could get back to work and be with his family. The plan was that

30

my daughter and my grandson would come to help when I got out of the hospital.

Marilyn had become disoriented. My nephew, Jeff, took her to the emergency room. A stay in a hospital care center followed. We believe she'd had a shock reaction to what was happening to me. I will not continue with her story, except to say she is fine now. I mentioned it only to acknowledge the added stress my son, daughter, and nephew had just acquired.

✳ ✳ ✳

Craig wrote that I sounded upset during his morning call to me. I proceeded to tell him there had been a big and very loud party going on outside my room the night before. I added that friends of ours (who lived quite far away) were celebrating a family wedding. Yes, right there in the ICU. (Poor Craig actually wrote about this concern of mine!)

Notes from Craig's 9:30am visit paint quite a different picture:

> **Craig's Notes**
>
> EASTER SUNDAY, APRIL 11
>
> I arrived at the hospital to find you sitting in a chair, watching TV. You told me that you got there mostly by yourself. You pulled yourself out of bed, took a few steps, and sat down.
>
> You also told me that you ate very well this morning. You are still on the oxygen mask and get tired very quickly, but "today is a new day" and things look much better.

My memory includes a verbal battle with Nurse Pam, my strong but encouraging day nurse. She had told me that today was a good day to get out of bed.

"So soon?" I'm pretty sure I wailed. "Do you realize how far down the floor is from the top of the bed? And the chair is sooo far away."

I have no idea how she convinced me to move to the edge of the bed, put my feet on the riser, and then drop down to the floor. I'm rather sure I needed a lot of verbal and physical help. I do know that for most of my stay in the ICU, I insisted I could not get out bed without wearing a breathing mask. Many times I was assured I did not need the mask. I usually got my way.

I learned later that people often have a hard time being weaned off oxygen. I think the mask became my "Dumbo's feather." It gave me courage. I felt safer when I wore it.

Once I was coerced into getting out of bed, I made the harrowing journey all the way across the twelve to eighteen inches that separated the bed from the chair. By the time Craig arrived, I was ready to take full credit for my bravery. As time passed, I would refer to that Easter Sunday as my rebirth.

Later, Pam insisted that Craig leave, in hopes I would get a two-hour nap. So much for a break for Craig. He filled his time off with going to my home to catch up on mail, messages, watering, and paying some bills. He was gone, but then returned within four hours.

After Craig and I went through my mail, I started my shake therapy. They strapped a black vest on me that vibrated like crazy to loosen the phlegm from my lungs. Quite an experience!

Whenever you go into a hospital, please have patience with the medical staff. They have to put up with some very sick and scared people. Long after I left the hospital, I became aware that I had not always been a sweet, soft-spoken ICU resident. Craig had had to remind me to be polite.

Craig's Notes

MONDAY, APRIL 12 (2nd week after the treadmill test)

When I came in, you were sitting in the chair. You looked well and said you felt good. You reported that last night was the first good night's sleep you've had in a while.

The cardiologists, hematologists, and others are trying to decide what else they want to do for you. They will probably recommend inserting an AICD.[1]

You seemed to like the idea of this "insurance policy" device.

Kristin said to tell you that Aengus, about ten months old now, gave his first real full wave to you while they were watching a video of you!

You worked very hard to finish your chicken at dinner,

---

[1] An AICD/ICD (Automatic Implantable Cardiac Defibrillator) is a device that constantly monitors heart function and kicks in if your heart stops beating.

> but we had to be creative by cutting it in very small pieces and adding, with each bite, some "gravy" that was actually your energy drink. Eating takes a lot out of you. You had enough energy, however, to recite a long list of tasks for me. I should be able to take care of most of them tomorrow.
>
> You said you feel like you are in good hands with Mike, the night nurse. He seems quite competent.

Are you noticing that I was just three days out of the induced sleep, doing quite well, and yet had developed quite a demanding nature? What was I doing to my son?

> **Craig's Notes**
>
> TUESDAY, APRIL 13
>
> Mike washed your hair. This was the first hair washing in over two weeks. You told me that Mike was "top-notch!"
>
> You walked the length of the bed, but are still quite breathless.
>
> They will take some fluid out from behind your right lung this afternoon. This should help your breathing significantly. You got a straw out of its paper wrapper today all by yourself, and told me, "Write it down!"

Conquering the straw: I can still see the breakfast tray with the milk in the waxy paper container and the straw beside it. I remember starting to roll the straw to the edge of the tray with what felt like a hand in a too-big-mitten .

I managed to get the straw between my two hands. I brought the straw to my mouth and tore off the tip of the paper with my teeth. I spit out the bit of paper and grabbed the straw with my teeth, while the useless fingers of my two hands held on to the rest of the wrapper. Success! I got the straw out of its wrapper. Then I just stared at the tightly closed milk box.

This time, I was overjoyed with my straw accomplishment. I honestly think I laughed, knowing there was no way I was going to open the milk container.

I guess I didn't starve to death. I'm here, aren't I?

> You keep exclaiming that you can't believe what a great team of people you have working to help you get better! You have mentioned a few times that you

> feel you are in such good hands.
>
> Current outstanding medical issues:
>
> • Fluid behind right lung
>
> • Lots of fluid still coming from the heart tube near your left lung
>
> • Urinary tract infection
>
> • Sore ("shark bites") on thigh from time when you had poor circulation and low blood pressure
>
> • Weak right hand, probably aggravated by a bad arterial line

Guinness, the therapy dog, came to visit.

> You were in an unbelievably good mood when I arrived. You stayed happy and strong the whole time I was there.
>
> You insisted on doing a bit of video to document this experience.
>
> We also wanted to make sure we remembered to write down the fact that, for some reason, everyone thinks you are a marathon runner! I told you to play along with that.

Craig reported that Nurse Michelle said she had initially heard "the runner story" from the doctors, and that it had been passed down from shift to shift. We still didn't know who started the rumor, but I suspected it might have been my primary care physician, Dr. Hauser. She must have told the other doctors that I had been working with trainers, and they must have equated trainers with athletic competitions. Not me. No sports.

When I'd retired, I'd decided to get more serious about my health. I tried to eat sensibly, but I was inconsistent with exercise. I had no self-discipline. Therefore, I had paid to have a trainer work with me.

Actually, by the time of the treadmill test, I had two trainers. I really was concerned that I wasn't getting stronger after my trip to Michigan.

Though Craig hoped I would play along with the doctors, just as he had been doing, each time a doctor said "I hear that you are a runner," I just had to giggle. "Me, a runner? Not even close."

✳ ✳ ✳

During Craig's early-morning visit on April 14th, Michelle told us a strange story about the night of my bypass surgery: She said she had felt compelled to go into my empty room when I was taken to the cath lab to check on my slow recovery. While she was there, she'd heard a little girl's voice calling her name.

Michelle had heard her own name called out four times that night. Arnold, another nurse, had heard his name called three times. On one occasion, Michelle and Arnold had heard each other's name being called.

Michelle asked me, "Who was that little girl?"

I was startled by both the story and the question. I assumed Michelle thought the voice came from a little girl I knew who had died. I told her that although I'd had a brother who had died before I was born, I couldn't think of any girl who would fit the story.

"I guess it was Grace," I finally said, referring to my very-much-alive three-year-old granddaughter. I felt we had a special bond, since she was my first granddaughter. We also shared the bond of being born in The Year of the Dragon, sixty years apart.

Much later, I asked Michelle whether that story was true. She assured me that it was. Then she added that she had called her mother to share the story. Her mother had not been shocked. She was a pediatric nurse, and often heard stories from her young patients about hearing voices or feeling someone's presence in their hospital room.

There is one last piece to the story: I was with my son's family about a year later. Out of the blue, my daughter-in-law said, "It couldn't have been Grace." It took me awhile to realize she was referring to the little girl's voice the nurses had heard in my ICU room.

The comment caught me off-guard. Assuming she meant the voice had come from an angel, I responded with the silly remark, "I guess I don't know the rules."

Her next question was, "Did you ever have a miscarriage?"

My jaw dropped, and then I said, "Yes."

In the early '70s I'd had an unplanned pregnancy that ended when the embryo got stuck in my fallopian tube (ectopic pregnancy). It was my first brush with death. The tube burst, and I was bleeding internally. My doctor said he'd almost lost me.

My baby would have been born in June, two years after Craig's birth.

Overcome with emotion, I called my daughter to tell her about this child, her unborn sister. I can't help but think that this child was with me the night of the bypass surgery. I think she was calling to the nurses to plead with them to not give up on me. My husband and I had even had a name ready during my pregnancy—Allison Michelle—in case we had a girl.

I'm grateful that my daughter-in-law offered such a beautiful explanation for the voices heard by the nurses the night of my surgery.

✳ ✳ ✳

Bit by bit, my strength was returning. Later that day, I was excited to tell Craig I had finally realized that the remote did not weigh fifty pounds. Those first days, I had been so frustrated when well-meaning attendants would move the remote out of the way and then forget to put it back close to me. I had very little strength, and reaching for the device that could connect me to a nurse felt like a struggle over rough terrain. By the time I finally captured the remote, pushing the button took my last burst of energy. I can still remember the feeling of panic the times when I could see it but couldn't reach it.

I was having a real problem ingesting enough food to get the nutrition I needed. We were told that the average ICU patient needed 3,400 calories a day just to maintain their weight. Tons of energy goes into the healing process.

I had to somehow get in six cans of an energy drink, plus orange juice with energy powder stirred in. At first, the chocolate or strawberry drinks had seemed to be a treat. But drinking six cans during or between meals every day was a tough job.

Just before Craig left I told him, "This has been the most interesting life experience!"

✳ ✳ ✳

The next morning, April 15th, I walked all the way down the ICU hall and back with Pam.

She told us I was now at the stage where I would probably get better each day. I was past the tenuous stage, she said, during which people may alternate three steps forward with one step back. Things were looking rosy.

6

Up, Down, Up, Down …

Craig wrote that he woke up on April 16th with Nurse Pam's good words buzzing in his head: "Your mother is now at the stage where she's likely to get better each day."

During Craig's early-morning call on the 16th, he was disappointed to hear that concern had been building through the afternoon of the day before. I'd lacked energy, had trouble breathing, and had shown signs of pneumonia setting in. Those unsettling symptoms had interrupted the talk of putting in the AICD, the heart-assisting device.

When Craig arrived he was asked to stay outside my room, where several doctors stood conferring about rectal bleeding. A tube down my nose ruled out a stomach problem. The issue was in the lower intestine, possibly ischemic colitis, which can arise when too little oxygen reaches the intestinal tissues. They wanted to "scope it," but decided to hold off, as tissue could tear, causing more harm than good.

I told my son, "Despite these setbacks, I'm happy that it's clear there's something else going on. I was afraid I was just being lazy, or not trying hard enough in physical therapy."

Craig's Notes

FRIDAY, APRIL 16

Today was a hard day for me. You were definitely weaker than yesterday, and since they won't let you eat for a while I assume you will keep getting weaker. This is disappointing, especially after Pam's comments about how you should just get stronger and stronger from now on.

Sitting in your room while you napped, it was hard on me to hear your moans and groans. You told me you

---

> were not in any pain, and the nurse said that moaning while sleeping is quite normal. Upon waking, you seemed to be happy and feeling good.

Craig stayed through the shift change. He left after he saw I was in good hands with the night nurse.

> **Craig's Notes**
>
> SATURDAY, APRIL 17
>
> So far, so good. A visit from the GI doctors ended with the news that the problem was not ischemic colitis. On the lining they found some small, quite normal polyps that appeared to have been irritated. They were probably bleeding because of the blood thinner drug, Lepirudin.
>
> Dr. Redfield, the infectious disease doctor, also liked what he saw. Okay. Things are looking up again.

Up, down, up, down, during this fairly mild phase of my roller coaster ride.

Craig's notes from Sunday, April 18th, say that I seemed much stronger. They were able to cut back on the oxygen. Yea!

Not so fast. Craig was paged as he dined with my nephew, Jeff, who was in town to celebrate his daughter's birthday. Dr. Jamil, a critical care doctor, informed Craig that the bleeding hadn't stopped. They were trying to find its source so they could stop the blood loss.

Up, down. Up, down. Up, down.

Nurse Elmer stayed with me the whole time. Just before 7:00pm, he told Craig they had found the "hole" and embolized it. I had required three pints of blood during the procedure. (Later, when I learned how much blood I had been given during my hospital stay, I felt better knowing I had been a regular blood donor for years.)

That evening the night nurse told Craig I was doing well, that all vital signs were good and I was resting. She said I had been given a lot of pain medications.

✳ ✳ ✳

At various stages, someone from my medical team would feel compelled to help Craig realize how limited my life might be once my condition stabilized. There was one point at which Nurse Pam had a serious talk with him. Pam had been the first nurse to encourage me to get out of bed and walk to the nearby chair. After a few setbacks she said, "Maybe it is time for you and your mother to realize that she may face a future of only being able to go from bed to a chair and back to bed."

My son quickly (and wisely) said, "Do not tell that to my mother!"

* * *

My memories are filled with my caring medical team laughing with me in the middle of my great adventure. I know there were scary times and painful procedures, but I seem to have chosen to block those thoughts.

As I began to share my funny stories, friends said, "You have to write these stories down."

* * *

Here's a story that did not make it into Craig's notes: During one of my groggier phases, I managed to pluck a hunk of hair out of my head. A nurse was coming into my room just as I raised my hand with the sprig of hair in it.

"Oh, don't do that!," she cried out.

Oops. Too late.

My hairstylist would later have the task of concealing that nickel-sized hairless circle behind my right ear.

You can laugh now. It's funny. I'm alive and I'm sitting here writing this stuff! That chunk of hair found a home in the scrapbook I later assembled.

* * *

I have described myself as being tightly wired. My mind dashes here and there. I over-think my own decisions and other people's comments. I have always been a rapid-fire talker, a nervous laugher, and, yes, a nail fiddler (not exactly a biter).

The moment the tube was removed from my throat after my nine days of deep sleep, I was more than ready to talk. As soon as Craig got in a few words about what had been happening, I started with a long and detailed account of my dreams.

It didn't take long for others to realize that talking wore me out quickly. Breathing was difficult. Nevertheless, whenever anyone entered my room I wanted to talk. I had no idea how sick I was. I would drift in and out of sleep while gazing at the TV screen. Anyone who came into my room was entertainment for me. Whether the person was emptying my wastebasket, bringing in my food tray, or performing some medical procedure, I always had something to say.

The doctors pleaded with my son to do whatever he could to get me to stop talking so much. They insisted I was using up too much energy. My body needed rest if it was going to heal.

I now know just how hard it was on Craig to have to be stern with me. One day he taped a sign with bold letters to the whiteboard:

> **EAT**
>
> **SLEEP**
>
> **DON'T TALK**

During one of her visits my daughter-in-law asked him, "Couldn't you have at least said 'TALK LESS?' "

The message did look a little harsh, but poor Craig had been caught between a rock and a hard place. He knew I enjoyed talking with everyone. He also knew the doctors needed his help to minimize my talking. Those who know me well understand exactly the perilous tightrope my son was attempting to traverse.

On another occasion I was offended when he said, "Don't forget to say 'Please' and 'Thank You.' " Why would he say that to me? I'm always nice to people. Ah, but you know. You've already read how bossy I was beginning to be to my son. It seems I was not always pleasant to the staff, either. I remember how upset I would get when I couldn't reach the remote for the television—the same remote that had the "Call Nurse" button. At first, when I lacked the strength to grab the heavy remote, it was scary to think I couldn't call for a nurse if I needed one.

✳ ✳ ✳

On a lighter note, Nurse Mike came up with several suggestions to make my recovery easier. Eating was a real challenge. Chewing seemed so difficult to manage. I'm sure the food wasn't tasty, since I was on a severely restricted low-salt, low-fat diet.

Seeing how long it took me to eat dinner, Mike suggested we ask the kitchen staff to puree my food. I told him I had grown up hiding my vegetables in mashed potatoes. Since I liked casseroles and stew, I thought it would be fine if they mixed my pureed meat and vegetables together.

We were delighted when my dinner tray arrived with unappetizing brownish-gray blobs of pureed meat and vegetables. My food may not have looked good, but it slid down more easily. With every spoon of food followed by a sip of my energy drink, mealtime became almost manageable.

✳ ✳ ✳

When Craig and my nephew, Jeff, arrived one morning I was sitting in a chair. I told them the doctors were pleased with my breathing. No recent scary sessions. I recall commenting that the gelatin, the energy drink, and the mango juice tasted divine!

✳ ✳ ✳

Hang on. We're heading up a steep hill. What comes after the crest?

Craig's Notes

MONDAY, APRIL 19—three weeks in the hospital

Dr. Nodurft, GI doctor, reported that they found the bleeding coming from an artery that feeds the rectum. Unfortunately, this area does not have many blood supplies, and stopping one could impact the function of the bowels six to twelve months down the road.

Hematologists came in and again described the delicate balance and the odds game they are playing by trading off clotting against bleeding. The working theory is that the clotting is Heparin-induced. (Heparin, a blood thinner used during bypass surgery, has been known in rare cases to clot blood instead of thinning it.)

This condition can last up to six months. They will want to keep you on blood thinners for at least that long. They are more concerned about the risk of clotting than about the risk of bleeding.

Jeff and I picked up Kristin from the airport and returned for a nice afternoon visit. You looked content and did an excellent job letting others speak, saving

---

> your energy. I know this was hard for you.
>
> 8:30pm: The night nurse said the bleeding was continuing at a low level. They will probably stop the Lepirudin.

The following day, poor Craig was again beset with contradictory messages. First he heard that the bleeding had slowed down. Then, Dr. Jamil paged him at work to tell me I had started bleeding badly again.

> **Craig's Notes**
>
> TUESDAY, APRIL 20
>
> The doctors are not enthusiastic about going through the arteries again because of the risk of probable long-term damage. They did a colonoscopy but did not find any obvious lesions.
>
> Mom's Dictated Notes for Today:
>
> "Last night I went to bed earlier, which made the night longer. There was a lot of chatter about 'We've got to get her down to the OR to find and stop that bleeding!' I asked, 'Have you called my son?' One doctor finally decided they should not operate because 'her rectum would die.' That was scary, but I went right back to sleep.
>
> "Guinness, the therapy dog, came to visit again today.
>
> "Kristin and Jeff visited. There was lots of cleaning up before they arrived, enemas and such. I was a good patient but did call out in pain a time or two. They apologized for all the careful scraping, explaining that they wanted to figure out 'this mystery down below.'"

Are you getting this picture? I was treating my son, who was dealing with my serious medical situation, as if he were my secretary. I hope I had some softness to my tone. I'm afraid I didn't. I was in my own small world, totally oblivious to the other obligations my son was juggling.

Craig wrote that Dr. Jamil said I was still the sickest patient in the ICU, mostly because of the clotting and bleeding risks. I wonder, should I be proud that I was finally the best at something?

> **Craig's Notes**
>
> WEDNESDAY, APRIL 21
>
> Kristin is here from Michigan. To keep Aengus on his normal routine, my sister decided to leave him with his daddy in Michigan. She is taking a shift at the hospital while I go and pretend to work at my job.
>
> You are having a quiet day. No sitting in the chair. Good breathing all day. Still a little bit of "lava flow." The hematologists have taken you off all blood thinners until further notice. Bob is your day nurse. You are in good spirits.

Liz came by to give me another relaxing Healing Touch session. What a gift!

As I read in a November 5, 2007, article in USA Today, "Healing touch is not a massage. Sometimes the practitioner's hands hover above the body and don't actually make contact. Healing touch is an 'energy therapy' that uses gentle hand techniques purported to help re-pattern the patient's energy field and accelerate healing of the body and mind. It is based on the belief that people have fields of energy that are in constant interaction with the environment around them … ."

Scripps Green Hospital began offering the treatment to open-heart surgery patients as far back as 2002. I believe that Healing Touch and guided imagery audiocassettes helped lessen my stress level.

I wish Liz could have worked her magic on Craig and Kristin!

In addition to visiting me and spelling Craig, Kristin planned to go to San Francisco to help Jeff with my sister's medical situation. Craig, Kristin, and Jeff were all being pushed to their limits. I had no idea until at least a year later of the sacrifices they were making for my sister and me.

I realize that they acted out of love, but I can't help feeling pangs of guilt once in a while. I know they do not want me to feel guilty about a situation that was out of my control. It's extreme gratitude for their love, encouragement, and emotional support that I feel most often.

7

Things Are Looking Up

Each day had its share of adjustments. For example, I had to learn how to sleep with an oxygen mask without lying on the air tubes.

They did a Doppler scan to look for blood clots. The clot in my right leg was growing. The critical care doctor told us they were thinking about inserting an IVC filter[1] to prevent the clot from moving to the heart or brain.

Best story of April 22nd: I wanted to use the commode in my room. No, not the one in the bathroom. The commode was just a potty seat on the floor, hidden behind a privacy screen.

Since walking meant dragging lots of wires, it was easier to walk to the potty seat than to the real toilet. My energy was nonexistent. I needed my nurse and a helper to move me from the chair to the potty. Those nine days in deep sleep, coupled with my many medications, had significantly weakened me. The muscles in my legs were shot.

Potty mission accomplished, I felt like a limp washrag.

Looking up at the top of my mountain-high bed, I realized there was no way my nurse was going to get me into it. Have I mentioned that I would have to step up on a platform to climb onto it? The task looked formidable.

Realizing I was dead weight, I shouted, "Go and get the biggest, burliest man you can find to help me get into bed."

The nurse's helper darted out of the room. I guess the message spread, because Tony came in. With no explanation, the nurse sent him away

---

[1] An IVC filter is a small metal device designed to prevent blood clots from traveling to the lungs. The filter is typically placed just below the kidneys, in the inferior vena cava (the large vein that takes blood back to the heart).

without letting him help. On his way out he grumbled, "What, I'm not big enough?"

I was thinking he should stay until another man arrived. Wouldn't it be easier for two guys to hoist me into bed? I felt like I weighed two hundred pounds.

Then big, strong, well-built Eric arrived to rescue me. You should have seen the muscles on that guy! I held on to him as if he were a big carnival teddy bear. I don't remember him picking me up, but he must have, because I'm pretty sure my legs were worthless. I think I swooned. As he left, I do remember thinking he smelled so good!

* * *

On Friday, Nurse Pam's special treat was to take me down the hall for a real shower.

That evening, Michelle told Kristin and Craig on the phone that the doctors had not inserted the filter because the clot had not progressed. They also learned that I had become tearful and requested a tranquilizer.

"She has a lot to deal with, and she's having a hard time coping today," Michelle said.

By the time they arrived after dinner, I was feeling better. The visit was long and joyful, highlighted by video clips of Grace, Tori, and Aengus. Seeing my grandchildren was priceless medicine.

* * *

Later, when my daughter became aware that I wanted to write about my medical journey, she shared some of her first impressions on seeing me in the hospital.

Kristin wrote, "Your legs were all puffy, like fat hot dogs. The pump that pulled fluid from your heart was scary looking—gory, actually."

On a happier note, she felt that the nurses and staff were super nice and "loved you." She had made a special connection with Michelle, whom she described as "awesome."

Do you recall that Kristin learned about my need for bypass surgery right after going out to her first movie since the birth of her baby? For years after that, she said, she was paranoid about going to movies as she associated movies with my illness.

* * *

During Michelle's night shift on Thursday, I had mentioned having missed a hair coloring appointment. "I'll be with you tomorrow night," she'd said. "Let me color your hair. I'll bring in a movie for you to watch on my computer while I work on your hair."

What could I possibly say? "Yes! Yes!"

Sure enough, Michelle arrived Friday night with hair care equipment and her computer. (I know she had other patients who required caring words, pills, bedtime washing, monitor checking, and so on. I hope the other demands on her were light that evening.)

I'm pretty sure it was close to 11:00 when she was finally free to become "hairdresser extraordinaire." She set up her computer first, so we could watch *Under the Tuscan Sun.*

I was treated like royalty! It felt wonderful to have a caring person gently massage my head and wash my hair. Hair coloring, trimming, styling, and girl talk gave me a huge morale boost. The romantic comedy was the best possible "chick flick" for our girls' night fun. The festivities ended about 1:30am, with Michelle walking through the halls inviting nurses to come see me and my pretty hair.

Can you imagine my surprise when Michelle offered to work with my hair? Are you able to feel the love I was developing for the medical staff? And not for just my medical team. Most of the people who came into my room, no matter what their task, were pleasant. They all commented on the poster with the photos of my grandchildren. My memories are filled with the warm, caring, funny people who were constantly challenged by my setbacks. We appreciated the compassion they displayed.

I began to refer to the hospital as "Scripps Green Hotel Royale." The purple latex gloves worn during most procedures added a luxurious touch. I saved an unused pair as a souvenir, along with a sample of the pretty paper placemats decorated with purple and soft-green flowers.

When Craig called the next morning I told him, "I have the greatest hairstyle ever." Michelle had already told him I'd started the day singing "Oh What a Beautiful Morning" from the musical *Oklahoma.*

* * *

Craig asked Michelle about my blood clots, and she told him they were in my calves. So far, they were not growing. Clots above the knee, we were told, can travel to the heart or lungs and cause a heart attack or pulmonary embolism.

On Monday morning, April 26th, four weeks after my treadmill test, the nurses reported that I was doing well. It was suggested that it might be time to insert the AICD.

They did an echocardiogram, after which I walked the full circle of the ICU with my physical therapist. What an achievement!

The following day all the doctors seemed to be feeling good about my progress, though they were concerned about my rectal bleeding. There was some discussion about doing plastic surgery on my leg when they inserted the AICD, which Dr. Rogers said would happen in a day or two.

There were several pieces of good news. My nutrition numbers were nearly normal, and the hematologists affirmed that no filter would be required to protect my heart and brain from blood clots. Best of all, Dr. Housman came in with a big smile to tell us the echocardiogram showed incredible recovery of heart function.

After a really good night's sleep, you would think I'd have been feeling relaxed and happy on Tuesday. I was, but I'm afraid I sounded a bit frustrated when I spoke to Craig on the phone. I just wanted to make sure everyone was communicating well before each decision and action. There were so many aspects to consider.

And consider they did. Dr. Redfield didn't want to take any chances with infection when they put in the AICD/pacemaker, so they decided they would put off that procedure and take care of the leg on Wednesday. I was glad they were paying so much attention to those details.

✶ ✶ ✶

I called Craig that evening to tell him I had hit the jackpot: Bonnie, of Finnish ancestry, was my night nurse! Bonnie had grown up in Wisconsin and had never been to Finland, but knew the language. And her best friend was from Ishpeming, Michigan, where a Finnish cousin of mine was born.

All four of my grandparents were born in Finland. They emigrated to the United States as adults. I told Bonnie about the House of Finland, which is part of the International Cottages in San Diego's Balboa Park.

After Bonnie had been my nurse a few times, she told me she wanted to adopt me. How sweet for someone younger than I am to say that.

✶ ✶ ✶

Remember when they said I would probably be in the hospital about five days? Four weeks had passed since the stress test I had requested and the "no-big-deal" bypass surgery. And all that time Craig had been taking his amazing notes, filled with specific details—the notes he had started so he could report accurately to Kristin.

As my condition zigged and zagged, the facts began to be augmented by interesting "people stories." I have to assume Craig knew I would enjoy learning the whole story someday.

How did I spend my time when I wasn't being fussed over? I was often drowsy. I remember watching a lot of TV. Drifting in and out, I would see the end of a show and then the beginning of a movie. I hardly ever saw anything from start to finish. I don't remember reading a book. I had lost the use of my hands for tasks like writing. I didn't have my cell phone in the hospital, and even if I'd had one, I'm sure I could not have placed a call or played solitaire on such a little gadget.

I became fascinated with my international medical team. Thus began my favorite activity. The staff wrote the names of my nurses and any info I needed to know on a big whiteboard in my room. I started to ask people who entered to write their name, their medical specialty, and their ethnic origin. I had always been proud of my Finnish ancestry. I hoped others would enjoy telling me about their backgrounds.

Craig began to make a list of the names and ancestral countries. By the time I left Scripps Green the list included some forty nations, plus three Native American tribes.

My personal favorite came from a male nurse who said his family believes they are descended from an African tribe. I think he said it was the Mandingo tribe in West Africa.

Even with the medical successes and setbacks to record, Craig took the time to include in his notes the bits of lightness as well as my bossy dictations. Could he possibly have guessed what a treasure he was preparing for me?

* * *

Craig's Notes

WEDNESDAY, APRIL 28

The good:

Walked the full ICU loop while only lightly holding on to someone's hand.

Nice phone conversation with just a little shortness of breath.

Ate a cheeseburger, specially ordered by Nurse Pam.

The not so good:

Looked quite tired while eating.

Walked only one-quarter of the way around ICU in the

---

afternoon.

Energy is slipping.

Dr. Schneider, the plastic surgeon, told me the surgery on the leg wounds, which has been put off until tomorrow, is not just cosmetic. They want to avoid future infection. It may require several skin grafts, done in stages. Future stages could be done after discharge.

Since Craig's notes from Thursday, the 29th, are lengthy, with reports from five doctors representing five different medical specialties, I will summarize some of that content here:

Suspecting that my shallow breathing might be due at least in part to blood clots, they decided to insert the IVC filter after all, perhaps a removable one. It seems that a quick drop-off of oxygen concentration during the previous afternoon's physical therapy session had added to the urgency of that procedure.

Then they got the idea to take me to the cath lab for a pulmonary angiogram, the gold standard for detecting clots. They said they wanted to do that before the plastic surgery on the leg, then changed their minds and decided to do the leg first.

There was a lot of back and forth, weighing the options. Then, based on input from Interventional Radiology, they decided to do a less invasive pulmonary CT scan first. If it came out positive for clots, they would implant the filter to prevent clots from reaching my heart or brain.

Shortly after noon they determined that it would be best to do the plastic surgery first. So off we went.

This may be a good time to tell about the sores on my right leg. Craig's notes barely mention what happened because the medical staff said very little on the subject. At this point I was aware of a gaping wound behind my right knee and another farther up on my right thigh. An earlier note had referred to oozing from one of the wounds.

I'm not sure when I was told what had caused the wounds. I became aware that the problem involved an Ace bandage on my right leg during bypass surgery. I understand it had been left in place too long after the surgery. This new complication had brought a new field of doctors into my medical team when the bandage finally came off and the wounds were exposed.

On a lighter note, Nurse Marsha told Craig she would think about what actress should play her role in the upcoming movie about this adventure. Looking back at Craig's notes now, I see a black-and-white silent movie with a cast of many doctors, followed by voluptuous nurses running in and out, crisscrossing each other's paths. Bouncy piano music fills the theater as the screen shows the words "I want to do my surgery first. Out of my way!" There were so many options it was sort of like a Keystone Kops comedy.

What a day! By the time they returned me to my room, after Dr. Schneider worked on my leg, Craig said all I could think about was wanting the biggest chocolate chip cookie they could find. He bought an obscenely supersized chocolate chip cookie from the vending machine outside. I devoured it with glee!

8

Medicine for Grandma

It's May. Will it be the Merry Month of May for me? Where are we now, and how did we get here?

- Treadmill stress test: 3/29, surprising results
- Angiogram: 3/30, bigger surprises, including silent heart attack
- Bypass surgery: 3/31, five bypasses hyperclotted; seven stents
- Induced sleep: 3/31 – 4/9; she's talking
- Amazing progress: through 4/15
- Up, Down, Zig, Zag: bleeding, clots, fluid, trouble breathing
- Yet to do: AICD, IVC filter, pull fluid, plastic surgery

On Saturday, May 1st, I had a sweet early-morning phone conversation with an almost-four-year-old Grace. She told me she loved me and missed me. Then she suggested, "When you're done being sick you can come over to stay at my house, and then I can come over to stay at your house." That certainly gave me an incentive to get the heck out of the hospital.

The Kentucky Derby was the big event that day!

In my typical fuzzy state I gazed at the TV. I was channel surfing when I heard bits about the famous race and the horses that would be racing. Since it was a Saturday, I had the double treat of having my son and daughter-in-law visit me.

Nurse Artene popped into my room with the news that the nurses were setting up a betting pool. "Would you like to place a bet?"

"Sure!" Craig offered to lend me money so I could participate. I bet on Smarty Jones, a horse whose name I had heard earlier on TV.

During the hours of pre-event interviews and reflections on past races, Craig treated me to a gentle head massage and my daughter-in-law gave me an oh-so-soothing foot rub. Just before the race was finally about to start, I heard a nurse going from room to room, warning, "This is your last chance to pee, get help sitting up, take medicine, or ask for fresh water.

The race is about to begin. For the next several minutes, no nurses will be available."

It wasn't long before I heard cheering from the nurses' desk, and possibly from other patients as well. I joined in with, "Go, Smarty, go!" The roar from the grandstands, the sound of the horses whizzing by on the TV screen, and the final call filled my ears.

Yes, Smarty Jones won the race! Soon after, Artene came in with the seven dollars I had won.

(Hmmm ... I'm not sure I've ever paid back the money I borrowed from my son.)

Smarty Jones went on to win the Preakness, the second of the Triple Crown races. I won two dollars on that race. There were high hopes, but Smarty Jones's winning streak did not include the Belmont race.

✶ ✶ ✶

On Sunday, Craig told me three-year-old Tori had awakened in the middle of the night and kept saying, "Medicine for Grandma. Medicine for Grandma."

Tori must have sent a telepathic message to Nurse Karen, because she called my son's home and suggested bringing the girls in to see me. She told them everything was okay, but that I was quite tearful.

The girls came to visit me in the hospital patio that afternoon. It was a nice, spirit-lifting visit. They were not scared, were well behaved, and put on a good show! Despite this pleasant visit, it was a tough day for all because of my weakness and shortness of breath.

Craig's Notes
SUNDAY, MAY 2
Dr. Grudko said he does not plan to pull fluid out of the left lung cavity today. There are several things going on related to your breathing, and this is just one. He'd rather not do anything that is not absolutely necessary. He will give you two units of blood to help build your strength.

On May 3rd, after five weeks in the hospital and no end in sight, I was still weak. It frightened me that I could hardly breathe. There was talk about starting an antidepressant.

Craig said he was pleased to see the formerly typical huddle of doctors outside my door on Tuesday. Based on the recent echo, my heart was still working fairly well. We were happy to hear that my lungs looked fantastic, according to Dr. Jamil. No change with blood clots. Yea!

As for spirit lifting, Guinness was especially comforting that day and didn't want to leave when Ralph said it was time to go.

I guess I must have slept soundly that night, because Craig said the night nurse did a good job of fending off the X-ray people when I was sleeping so well. She also washed my hair on Wednesday morning.

Craig's Notes

WEDNESDAY, MAY 5

Dr. Rubenson restarted you on a medicine that helps the heart beat a bit stronger, and on a diuretic to keep the fluids coming out.

The plastic surgeon came in and said the wounds are healing nicely. They may elect to close them fairly soon.

Thursday was better than Wednesday, just as Wednesday had been better than Tuesday. I walked out of my room to the elevators and back—perhaps forty feet. Good news, yes, but don't forget that two weeks earlier I had walked three times that distance.

Craig's Notes

FRIDAY, MAY 7

I came in at 11:00am to find them preparing to take you to Interventional Radiology to implant the clot filter. This bothered me significantly, as it was the first time a decision like this had been made without informing me.

I also understand that they will be implanting the permanent style rather than a removable one.

Their plan to insert a filter seems reasonable. Basically, what changed was, 1) they saw a change and growth in clots in the leg, and 2) echocardiograms performed today and yesterday showed increased pressure on the right side of the heart. They believe this could have been caused by small clots that have gotten to the heart. Also, based on those echoes, they believe that if a new clot did get to the heart, a bad heart attack would result.

All parties seem to be in agreement regarding installing the filter. The explanation for using a permanent

---

> filter is simply that all parties involved just don't have enough experience with the removable type to have confidence in it. They feel it is still in the experimental stage of development.

Craig said I looked good when he arrived, and I told him I had surprised myself by eating well and walking all around the unit. Even after the filter implant, I told him I considered this a good day. I told him I felt I was breathing better.

He said he'd raised a bit of hell trying to get some answers and letting people know that he was disappointed he hadn't been informed about taking me to Interventional Radiology to implant the filter.

"Damned if there weren't four doctors right here ready to explain things to you and me within a few minutes," he wrote in his notes. "Hee hee hee—we let them know who's boss, didn't we, Mom?"

Craig was dealing with another dilemma that involved a one-year assignment in Singapore with his company. Long before this hospital saga began, Craig had signed on to the project. The whole family was supposed to leave in a short time. At the time of my bypass surgery, the trip had seemed far off in the future. As my recovery dragged on, however, with its frequent complications, final decisions as to when and even whether they could leave were up in the air.

> **Craig's Notes**
> SATURDAY, MAY 8
>
> I called early in the morning to check with Nurse Jo. She told me you had cried before going to sleep. She said she had talked with you about how you have a right to feel sad, but that you are making slow, steady progress.
>
> After speaking with Jo, I asked to speak with the lead nurse about requesting the cheerleading type of nurse, like Jo, to help you recover at this stage. She said she would see what she could do.

It was a pretty good morning. I'd had a good breakfast and had walked over to take a shower. I was overjoyed when Craig arrived at noon with a sinfully rich Peanut Butter Cup Blizzard!

> During my telephone updates I spoke with Sally, Mom's college friend. When I told her about the breathing issues she brightened up and informed

> me that she had had her own episode of breathing
> difficulty recently and therefore could vouch for what
> Sally had to say:
>
> It turns out that we as a species are poor at breath-
> ing. Especially as we get older, we fall into a habit of
> horribly inefficient "chest breathing." Chest breath-
> ing is when your chest inflates and your shoulders
> move up.
>
> "Abdominal breathing" is much more effective at
> bringing oxygen into the body. Put your hand on your
> belly and breathe so that your belly inflates instead of
> just your chest. Then practice, practice, practice!
>
> When she got to the panicky state because of chest
> breathing, she said, she would concentrate on ab-
> dominal breathing and feel better almost immediately.
>
> She suggests that this is an important thing to
> work on, because healing is closely related to oxy-
> gen levels.

Can you imagine Craig taking the time to write out all that information about breathing?

I already knew all about deep, relaxing breathing. I would instruct
myself to relax my shoulders and breathe, and within seconds my shoulders would be back up by my ears. I worked hard at trying to relax, I really
did. But working hard and trying to relax canceled each other out.

I think I was more aware of my medical condition at this stage. I
remember the funny and sweet stories, but I think I was getting scared I
might not get better.

> **Craig's Notes**
> SUNDAY, MAY 9
>
> Seemed like a good day all around. There was one
> issue with blood oozing from your leg wound during
> your morning walk. Several doctors came to check,
> but everyone said it was good, natural healing of the
> wound.
>
> We brought Grace and Tori at about 1:00pm for a
> nice visit in the patio.
>
> Eating is still difficult, and it has become almost
> comical how often the nutritional drink comes. You
> filled out your own menu. I am happy you had a good
> weekend and look forward to a good week.

I had a wheelchair, but I was allowed to walk most of the way from my room to the patio. I think it was good for the girls to see me walking. I can see Grace setting down her backpack. Then she pulled out pieces of equipment for checking my heart, wrist, and legs. The charming two- and three-year-olds put on a sweet show for the passers-by.

Craig's Notes

MONDAY, MAY 10—six weeks in the ICU

You walked to the shower but had to be wheeled back to bed because of oozing from your leg. You ate fairly well, but still seemed kind of slow and lethargic.

Dr. Rubenson affirmed that you seemed to have less energy, and put you back on the medications you did well on last week. He said they had been changed on Sunday for some reason.

Dr. Schneider came in to look at the leg. He said not to worry about the oozing. He and a nurse decided to start "vaccing" the sores surrounding the wound and using a vacuum to clean it out. This promotes closing and healing. It can be done in concert with other procedures.

On Wednesday, Craig wrote that although I still seemed weak, I seemed to be breathing a bit better.

Craig's Notes

WEDNESDAY, MAY 12

Dr. Sinclair said you are stable and improving. They pulled off some fluids.

The fact that your breathing was better last weekend when there was less fluid gives weight to the theory that the fluid is the main contributor to the breathing difficulty.

Nancy, the wound care nurse, came in to "vac" your leg wounds. This involved putting a piece of foam in the wounds, sealing the area with tape, then applying the vacuum. This may be all that is needed to take care of the leg wounds; "closing" or skin grafts may be unnecessary. She said we would probably see a noticeable difference by Friday.

I stopped by to speak with Chris (ICU nurses' main supervisor) about getting cheerleaders assigned to you. I also mentioned that greater consistency might

---

help. I reminded her that you have had forty-four different nurses so far.

My son must have been feeling relief. He wrote that Thursday was a pretty good day, that I seemed to have much more strength, and was eating and breathing better.

Craig's Notes

THURSDAY, MAY 13

The theme for today was to take more control. This was motivated by yesterday's physical therapist, who said that walking is crucial. Besides the PT, nurses or family members can walk you, he said.

We devised our own in-room exercise routine, which involved getting up from one chair, taking a few steps, and sitting down in another. You did this eight times and surprised yourself by getting up from the chair without assistance.

We also called Kristin and Marilyn instead of waiting for the phone to ring.

Dr. Rubenson came in at about 6:00pm. He said he was happy with the change of meds, which seemed to be effective at getting rid of fluids. He also said that he thought your X-ray looked better. The strategy will be to stay the course through the weekend, then possibly implant the AICD next week.

Craig's notes make it clear I was getting very tired of being in the ICU! Yes, I'm sure I was. It cramped my style!

Craig's Notes

SATURDAY, MAY 15

I think today you were at your strongest yet. You walked around the unit three times, sat in the chair several times, and even had a bit of an appetite.

You called me at home in the evening to tell me you still felt strong and that it was still a good day. You also wanted to tell me about a special visitor.

I was jolted awake in the afternoon by a nurse, who burst into my room and crossed over to open my drapes. "You like music, don't you?" she asked in a loud voice.

My quick agreement brought the explanation that a woman would soon come to my room to play the violin for me. Just as the nurse was leaving my room I called out, "Wait! Can you find someone to use my video camera to capture this interesting memory for me?"

You probably know a patient's valuables are kept in a hospital safe. I, however, had my video camera sort of hidden in a cabinet near my bed. Sure enough, in came a staff member to get my camera and prepare to tape the surprise concert.

Seconds later, a lovely woman arrived and began to play beautiful music for me. I was entranced.

I learned later that the woman was First Chair Violinist with the San Diego Symphony. She had been a patient in this hospital with a long stay in the ICU many years earlier. On concert days the symphony would rehearse in the morning. During the time between the rehearsal and the concert, she would share her talent with patients in the hospital.

I may have been in a hospital setting with my health in flux, but I was treated with respect, compassion, and humor. Talk about making the best of a bad situation!

Craig's Notes

SUNDAY, MAY 16

You were not as upbeat today but seemed to be just as strong. You walked around the ICU three times before noon!

You told me Nurse X the Second was the night nurse. It had taken three call-button rings to get a bedpan. When she did come in, you said, she had explained that she didn't understand why you needed her help because she had heard you were walking around.

After a few other similar incidents, you said, "You don't know anything about me, do you?"

She had specifically told you that she had two other patients and not to bother her. "Don't ring the call button for every little thing."

I can always count on my son to find the silver lining in the face of adversity. Craig wrote that this unpleasant experience did not seem to set me back, unlike similar experiences I'd had. He made sure she would never be my nurse again. Three cheers for Craig!

> **Craig's Notes**
>
> TUESDAY, MAY 18
>
> I spoke with Dr. Grudko. He said things seem to be working. The plan is to slowly adjust the medicines that help the heart beat with more strength over the next few days. He said Dr. Rubenson is out of town for the week. The team doesn't want other cardiologists coming in to see you and changing the strategy while he is gone. He said you may be permanently crippled because of all that has happened to your heart. He hinted that Dr. Rubenson may have other ideas.
>
> Dr. Sinclair was a bit more positive than Dr. Grudko. She said you looked much better than you did on Friday. She also mentioned that the most recent echo showed an improvement.
>
> The AICD won't go in this week because they want you even stronger. They want Dr. Rubenson back in town when it is inserted.
>
> I spoke with you and Nurse Marsha around 6:30pm, and you both said the day was great. You ended up walking a total of four times today—two times when you were only holding on to someone's arm.

On Wednesday, Marsha was my nurse again—three days in a row! We were on a roll. And then on Thursday, I had her again! Craig wrote that I was fairly weak, which he figured might be due to the juggling of the heart medicines.

> **Craig's Notes**
>
> THURSDAY, MAY 20
>
> When I arrived at 9:45am, I saw something I had never seen before: No tethering to an IV pole! Besides that, your blood pressure was 124. Marsha said that they had been successful at getting fluids off again.
>
> I spoke with Dr. Sinclair at 11:30. She proudly proclaimed that you were totally off the heart-strengthening medicine and doing well. She also mentioned that they had started talking to you about going to a rehab center next week. There are a lot of things to consider, but just the fact that they are talking about this seems to be a big step forward.
>
> You walked around the unit and ate most of your lunch.

Craig came in on Monday with a slice of pizza for me, and I ended up
eating the whole "super slice." What would he think of next to cheer up his
mom?

Craig's Notes

MONDAY, MAY 24—eight weeks in the ICU

You were lazy for most of the morning, but otherwise
fine. I noticed that your oxygen saturation levels were
lower than they had been (low 90s, high 80s vs.
mid to high 90s). Nurse Laura noticed this also. She
spoke with Dr. Sinclair and ended up increasing your
diuretic to get you to pee off more fluids. This seemed
to work well.

It's becoming more clear that when there are fluids
you are lazy, tired, and out of breath. When the fluids
are not there, everything improves!

After your afternoon nap, Laura took you outside
and bought you coffee. You walked a lot of the way. I
spoke with you when I called at 6:00pm. You sounded happy.

The plan for the AICD is to put it in later on Wednesday. The OR is booked up tomorrow. Dr. Rubenson
and a lung doctor debated about fluids around the
lungs. Rubenson really wants to pull more off. They
may tap the fluid if the ultrasound, which will happen
tomorrow, indicates that there is a significant amount
there to pull off.

I was feeling good, even a little cocky as I rounded the last corner
of the ICU loop pushing an empty wheelchair for balance. Applause and
encouragement greeted me as I passed the nurses' desk. The next thing I
heard was Nurse Edwin's taunting, "Why don't you give me a ride?" So I
did. I gave him the ride of his life, for about two feet!

You had a nice visit with Guinness, your favorite therapy dog, who jumped up on the bed with you.

We met Peggy, Blue Shield's "high-intensity case
manager" today. She will help get you into the right

> rehabilitation facility and will follow your case through rehab and back home.
>
> They took you down to Interventional Radiology to tap fluid in the late afternoon. Laura told me they took off over a liter from the right side! Unfortunately, they think they may have introduced air into that space, which is not good. (Why must every procedure include a complication??)
>
> Dr. Jamil read a follow-up X-ray and told me later that the air is not expanding and they did not need to put in a chest tube. She'll keep an eye on it and call me if anything goes wrong. You are still on track for the AICD implant tomorrow morning.

A nurse showed me the vessel containing the fluid they had sucked out of me. It had an interesting shape. I asked whether I could keep it.

Later, my daughter said, "Mom, tell me you didn't keep the fluid." No, I didn't. I just got the cleaned-out vase. For many years I kept it in my bedroom to remind me that I had survived my medical challenge of 2004.

Craig had a long talk with Dr. Rubenson about my current status and possible future.

> **Craig's Summary:**
>
> Dr. Rubenson's answers assume a fairly close to best-case scenario. The strategy is to give you a chance to fly, outside of the hospital. Allowing for bumps along the way, we will know a lot more after you have been out for a month or so. You will either take off and do very well or you will look sick at rehab and have to come back to the hospital.
>
> If that happens, we will have to start talking about plan B.
>
> He likes the scenario of 1) hospital, to 2) rehab, to 3) living with us, to 4) living independently again.
>
> Regarding our trip to Singapore, a good plan would include all parties feeling comfortable through the living-at-our-home stage. Then we would set up the transfer to living with someone else or living on your own. This is certainly still a possibility before August, when my family should leave for our one-year assignment.

9

Setback!

Craig's Notes

WEDNESDAY, MAY 26—Setback (estimated at about one week)

I'm pissed! Upon arrival at 10:00am the nurse told me the AICD was cancelled because of air in the lung cavities.

In addition, you seemed miserable and started mumbling to me about what happened yesterday and this morning. You mentioned a lot of pain, needing to go to the bathroom, and hunger. You seem worse than I've seen you in weeks.

During a nap you seemed highly agitated. You were mumbling, and seemed to be searching for something with your left hand. I asked you whether you needed anything. You woke up easily and said you were fine, oh, except for the caterpillar crawling up your chest. I straightened your blanket, and you told me that it was okay now because I'd smooshed him.

Caterpillar? Craig reported some interesting things I said that day! Among them, he wrote that I told him I was talking about umbrellas and asked him whether he had any idea why, and he said no, he didn't. Caterpillars and umbrellas . . . maybe the umbrellas were for the caterpillars?

When you wake up and someone asks you whether you are okay, you generally say you are fine and ask whether you've been sleep talking again.

The air they put in your lungs is called a 20% pneumothorax on the right side, meaning that twenty percent of the right chest cavity is filled with air and the lung is collapsed by that amount. They don't want to insert the AICD because that goes on the left side, and they don't want to risk compromising the breathing on that side, too.

> This morphine day was very difficult for me. I hope you didn't have as hard a time as I did.

Craig's Notes

THURSDAY, MAY 27

You are much better today. We would like to believe what Dr. Grudko told us, namely that this air-around-the-lungs setback should not affect your overall recovery time. It just affects the timing of the AICD. You were coughing more, but I think that is supposed to be a good thing after this procedure.

You called us at home around 8:00pm to tell us you had a good afternoon and wanted to call Kristin. We decided it would be best if she called you. She did so, and it was a good conversation.

You also told me that maybe I didn't need to hang around quite so much. "Why don't you go surfing?" you suggested.

Ready for a story? The wound vac is an interesting piece of equipment. I think I was told that it was first used just a year or two before I needed its service. Its job was to gently pull out bits of dead tissue within the wound. I'm sure I was given a complete explanation of what it is and how it works.

During one of my super-groggy naps, I heard what I thought were motorcycles racing around the Torrey Pines Golf Course just outside and below my window. There was a loud roar, and I pictured grass and plants being uprooted. When Craig arrived I shouted, "Look out the window. Can you see motorcycles racing around down there? They will ruin the golf course. Somebody has to stop them!"

Craig calmly assured me that the noise was coming from the wound vac. I soon got used to the sound of the motor as it went on and then off for short periods of time. I don't remember how long a "cleansing session" lasted.

Craig's Notes

FRIDAY, MAY 28

The black fingertip is not black anymore! (This is one thing the hematologists were quite interested in. It showed up during the initial induced sleep time. It looked like the end of your finger was dead.)

You did well with exercise.

> **Craig's Notes**
>
> SATURDAY, MAY 29
>
> I think you are as strong as ever today. One of the doctors remarked that because you are continuing to slowly improve, you don't take as long to recover from setbacks.
>
> Per Dr. Rubenson's suggestion, I mentioned the AICD scheduling on Tuesday to anyone who would listen. Everyone seems to know that this is the plan, including Dr. Curtis, who does the scheduling. It looks like we are in good shape for this procedure to happen early in the week.
>
> You walked once before I arrived, then again after I showed up. During that second walk, you took two trips around the unit. That may have been the first time you have done that.
>
> I also brought you a cheeseburger kids' meal (including a Shrek 2 toy) with a strawberry shake. You had mentioned this craving. You said it tasted so GOOD!

Craig's notes from the next day show that I was still looking and feeling strong. He wrote that they'd been told my pneumothorax was "clinically not an issue." He explained that although there still might be some air in there, it wasn't enough to matter. My kids must have felt so relieved! He said they were happy to hear that I was doing so well that the only real reason I was still in there was to wait for the AICD implant.

> **Craig's Notes**
>
> MONDAY, MAY 31—Memorial Day, nine weeks in the ICU
>
> I'm pretty down today. You seem to be doing well, though you don't seem as strong as yesterday. You were sleeping when I arrived and were active during your sleep, including lots of mumbling and hand motions.
>
> They took you down to radiology to get a good-quality X-ray to make sure everything was okay before the procedure tomorrow. They reviewed the X-ray and things look good.
>
> I was a little disturbed later in the day when I called to speak with Nurse Artene. She said you were doing well and had slept quite a bit in the afternoon after I left. Then she said you had requested that the phone

> be put near you, since "Craig hadn't been by yet today." I really hope these drugs and this experience are not affecting your mind.

On Tuesday morning, Craig received a call at work from Nurse Anne, saying the AICD procedure was scheduled for noon. When he called at 7:15 and asked to speak with the day nurse he was instructed to call later because the nurses were "in report."

He said that would be fine, and asked who was caring for me. And . . . the woman told him it was the person we'd renamed "Nurse X, The Banana Thrower"!

Oh #*&@^#! After getting over being angry, he called back to speak with the lead nurse. It was Artene and, bless her soul, she told him she had changed the assignment to Anna.

Close call!

> **Craig's Notes**
>
> TUESDAY, JUNE 1
>
> I spoke with Dr. Sinclair on the way in. She said you looked and seemed to be doing well this morning. She also said two different X-rays had shown that your pneumothorax is completely resolved! She told me Dr. Rubenson had been speaking with the anesthesiologist and others about ways to minimize the trauma and invasiveness of today's procedure. For instance, they may try to NOT put you on a ventilator. We all have our fingers crossed for a good day.
>
> They came to get you at 11:30 and took you into the operating room at noon. You were VERY sleepy. I tried but couldn't wake you up when Guinness came in for his weekly visit. You woke up slightly during the ride down to the operating room and seemed to know where you were and what was happening. I really don't know why you seemed so sedated. Anna said you got something for nausea that was probably the result of taking all your meds with no food.

Craig wrote that I told him I had an interesting story for him, and that he told me he had one for me, too, and that it was probably about the same thing, Nurse X. And so it was.

> Anyway, I hope this super-sleepy state you are in is not a problem.

Dr. Rogers, cardiologist, came into the waiting room at 1:30pm, after the AICD was inserted, and said that everything had gone well. There was one component of the procedure he decided not to do, which involved implanting a wire that would pace both sides of the heart rather than just one. They had mentioned before the procedure that threading this particular lead was often complicated and sometimes so difficult that instead of threading it through one of the arteries, they do it externally.

Dr. Rogers decided not to even try to put in this wire because of the risk of doing so and, more importantly, because your baseline EKG did not indicate that you needed it. He also mentioned that if a future cardiologist decides you needed the feature to pace both sides of the heart, the device can be upgraded at that point. I liked this decision to minimize the procedure and told him so.

They also did not put in the large ventilation tube. Your oxygen saturations did drop, but they introduced only a small tube in your mouth and that was sufficient. I think this was another example of decisions and special precautions taken specifically for you, given your history. You will go back up to the ICU after recovery, in an hour or so.

You arrived back in your ICU room at 2:30pm. You looked more awake than before the procedure, with a big smile on your face.

The next morning, Craig wrote, my nurse said I was completely stable and doing well.

However, he said I made no sense when he tried to speak with me on the phone, that I mumbled a lot and sounded drowsy. He attributed that to the pain medication. It really knocked me out, and made me feel loopy.

Craig's Notes

WEDNESDAY, JUNE 2

They decided not to redo the wound vac today, but Nurse Nancy said the wound looked great.

After a lot of thought, I decided to go to the Padres game with my co-workers. I was surprised to see Nurse Artene there.

I saw you after the game, and you still seemed drowsy and loopy. Dr. Sinclair said you seemed fine during the day, but were probably having a slow recovery day after the surgery yesterday.

They did start the blood thinner Coumadin today. To avoid a possible complication of clotting with the Coumadin, they started administering Lepirudin this afternoon. They will watch carefully for the next few days.

If any bleeding or other negative indications occur, therapy will stop and anticoagulation will be ruled out for a while. Perhaps they would try again in six months. It could be successful in the future because the body retains the antibody from the Heparin condition for six to twelve months. If therapy stops, you will not have the extra safety net of thin blood.

Craig must have felt like I was about to be released from the ICU, because on Thursday he checked out Sharp Hospital Rehabilitation Center. He wrote that he was impressed.

Craig's Notes

FRIDAY, JUNE 4—nine and a half weeks in the ICU

You were transferred to 3 West, the regular part of the hospital.

Did you get that? I was leaving the ICU!

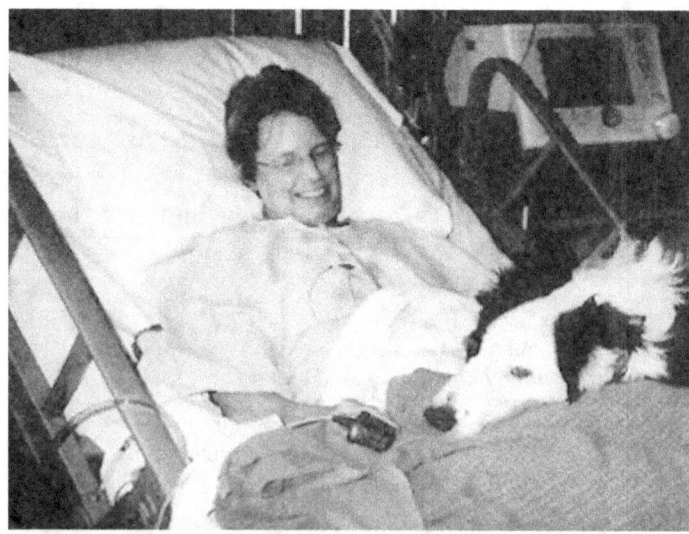

Guinness the therapy dog, my weekly visitor

> They had to stop the Coumadin because of rectal bleeding. They had hoped to have this safety net. They were not too disappointed though and said perhaps they'll try again in six months.
>
> I brought in margaritas to celebrate leaving the ICU. Nurses Pam and Melanie, as well as tall Ryan, your PT, each had one to help you celebrate.

Okay, Craig brought in margarita mix. But where was the tequila?! What? No salt?

I don't remember much about my new room. I was still in a hospital gown, but was not tethered to any equipment. I was finally able to get out of bed and walk to the bathroom alone without dragging a rolling pole. What a sense of freedom! I must have realized I was on a new section of my road to recovery. The doctors would not have let me leave the ICU unless they felt I was ready. Right?

I was nervous. I was weak and afraid to walk even a few steps without someone watching over me. It was reassuring to know that oxygen was available if I felt I needed it.

Sunday, June 6th, brought a visit from Jason, a close family friend. Then, for the first time, my granddaughters came into my hospital room. Their mommy and daddy had brought them to see me before, but only in the patio. Seeing them inside my room was another sign of my improving health. There was no stopping me now!

Monday, June 7th was pack-up-and-leave day. We heard moderately good reports from several doctors. The clot situation looked good. Dr. Grudko told Craig that the last echo result had been 35%, indicating that I had a stable though serious heart condition and was ready for rehabilitation. Craig's notes showed no further explanation of the 35%.

Echocardiograms (echoes) had been taken throughout my hospital visit, but neither Craig nor I had heard a result mentioned in the form of a percentage.

At 3:00pm the ambulance came to transfer me to Sharp Memorial Hospital Rehabilitation Center.

✳ ✳ ✳

I want to share a few thoughts on my stay at Scripps Green Hospital.

Guinness the therapy dog and his handler, Ralph, visited me every week. Their first visit came just four days after I came out of the induced sleep. Ralph and Guinness sat quietly by my bed that day. I doubt I was able to pet Guinness on that visit.

Each week, Ralph told me more about his dog. He said Guinness seemed to know when it was a visiting day. He even enjoyed the bath he had to have before he could enter the hospital.

Ralph took Polaroid photos of me with Guinness during many of the visits. Each week I would interact more with the dog. The highlight was the last visit, when Guinness was allowed to get into the bed with me.

There was one time when Ralph said they wouldn't be able to visit the next week. "We will see you in two weeks. Oh, you should be gone by then." When the two weeks passed, there I was, waiting eagerly to pet Guinness and talk with Ralph.

The therapy dog program is so good for patients. You already know I am a hyper person, tightly wired. I had tried meditation. I just couldn't turn off my mind. When Guinness was with me time slowed down, and so did my breathing—benefits similar to those available from meditating. Being with Guinness also reminded me of our family dog's abundant love and patience for each of us. He'd been the go-to body when any one of us was feeling down.

I assume that not all patients accepted Ralph's gift, but those who did received some of the best medicine the hospital could provide.

✳ ✳ ✳

My stay at Scripps Green Hospital was long and complicated.

The fatigue I had felt since my drive to and from Michigan did not seem to be fatigue in the classic sense. I never once thought my lack of energy or the breaking down of my knees and ankles had anything to do with my heart.

To add to the strangeness of my case, Judy, a college friend, reminded me weeks after my hospital stay and rehabilitation that one week before my treadmill test we had walked all over Wild Animal Park (now San Diego Zoo Safari Park).

"Really?!" I exclaimed. "Did we feed the giraffes?"

"Yes," she confirmed.

The giraffes were in the area known as The Heart of Africa. We would have had to traverse a long, fairly steep road to enter that area.

"Was I huffing and puffing on the steep grade?"

She answered, "Not that I remember."

I will never understand how my badly damaged heart had managed to function so well. I will be eternally grateful that I finally got the medical attention I needed. Thank goodness I had read the magazine article that encouraged women in their sixties to request a treadmill stress test!

When the angiogram revealed three badly blocked arteries and one totally blocked artery (silent heart attack), bypass surgery became the next logical step. My good overall health meant the chance of complications during surgery was in the one- to two-percent range, we were told. But ordinary surgery became un-ordinary when bypasses hyperclotted, necessitating the insertion of stents.

Though there was no one-hundred-percent proof, the working theory was that the clotting of my bypasses was due to an unusual clotting condition that can arise with the use of Heparin. Lepirudin, another of my anticoagulant drugs, led to bleeding every time we hoped to protect me from developing blood clots that could get to my heart or brain. Just before I left the hospital, my doctors wanted to introduce Coumadin, yet another widely used drug for thinning blood and preventing the formation of blood clots.

I do not believe my medical team could have foreseen my adverse reaction to Heparin. Since the drug is known to stay in your system for about six months, it most likely played a role in some of my setbacks.

The night before the surgery, my son and I had been given an anticipated timeline for surgery and recovery:

Anticipated time	**My Case**
Bypass Surgery: 2 1/2 to 4 hours	6 hours 40 minutes
Stents . . . unexpected	7 stents inserted
Induced sleep . . . unexpected	9 days
Total time in ICU: 1-2 days	66 days
Total Time in Hospital: about 5 days	69 days

＊ ＊ ＊

You might be interested to learn that my cousin Bill had quadruple bypass surgery the same year I had my surgery. While I was in the hospital he entered a different hospital, had his surgery, went into the ICU, was discharged, and got in some golf, all according to the normal anticipated timeline—while I experienced the unusual complications that extended my stay.

I am aware that the readers of my story will contemplate their own medical good or bad experiences and horror stories they have heard about what goes on in hospitals. Some may wonder why my family and I did not react more negatively during my many setbacks.

During the early stages my family was relieved when there was any sign that I would pull through the nightmare. While my progress was slow and erratic, interesting stories began to emerge once I came out of the induced deep rest. Humor slid into any little opening it could find. Kindness, compassion, encouragement, and clear communication with my son and me were noticed and greatly appreciated.

Months and years later, when someone expressed doubt or disdain about the care I'd received, my son reminded me, "Mom, they kept you alive." We were grateful the medical team had not given up on me.

I am pleased that my son did his best to remain positive in his thinking. He helped me stay strong when I became discouraged. He, like me, is more likely to give the benefit of the doubt, rather than rant and rave, when something doesn't make sense to him.

I am convinced that a big part of the reason I came through my ordeal unscathed and able to function so well physically and emotionally had to do with my son and daughter doing what they could to be sure the atmosphere surrounding me remained positive and encouraging.

It was about a year after my bypass surgery that I began to be fully aware of the stress my son and daughter had experienced as my heart problems played out. Relatives and other caretakers seldom get the emotional or physical support or the appreciation they deserve for easing the challenges of patients in or outside of hospitals.

While I was in my own world, hurdling the medical bumps, I received a lot of attention. I was also under the influence of drugs, in a bit of a haze. My son's notes remind me of my slow progress and emotionally painful setbacks. Friends and family members saw my bouts of tears and moments of pain, to which I have occasional flashbacks.

10
I'm Wired to Go Off!

It was at least a year after I left the hospital that an ICU nurse told me I had been showing signs of giving up. My medical team had gone into high gear, adjusting my meds and moving ahead with the insertion of a pacemaker and defibrillator (AICD).

Several times since April 11th my son had been told I would have the necessary procedure, only to hear of another postponement due to a new medical complication. The AICD was inserted ever so carefully on June 1st. I finally had the safety net of a device that could monitor my heart and jump-start it if the beating stopped.

Monday, June 7th, was my day to be transferred to Sharp Memorial Rehabilitation Center. First, I had to get out of my hospital gown and put on comfortable clothes—my own clothes, for the first time since March 29th! I was transported by ambulance, with my son following in his car.

New medical facility, new medical personnel, new expectations and activities awaited me. Did they fully understand the complications I had experienced? Would they help me move forward, but not too fast? I was not immune to new setbacks. I had not been given a clean bill of health. My sense of humor and positive attitude were being tested.

Semi-settled into my new room, it was time for me to give my ever-present, strong, tender, and compassionate son a goodbye hug. Within minutes a nurse came in with a hospital gown. As she helped me take off my T-shirt, she stared at my chest and burst out laughing. "WHAT IS THAT?!" she asked.

Tipping my head down as far as I could, I saw a strange sight. "I have no idea!" A large bandage covered the space between my breasts. Sticking out of the bottom of the bandage were two clear cylinders, somewhat larger than AA batteries, three and a quarter inches long and half an inch in diameter. Pulling back the bandage revealed purple caps on the cylinders.

Two orange wires stuck out of one tube, and two white wires protruded from the other. The opposite ends of the wires were inside me.

Peering into the tubes, we saw metal needles at the ends of the four wires. "Oh, my gosh! I'm wired to go off!" So much for being nervous in my new surroundings. My nurse and I bonded immediately as we howled with laughter. When she managed to catch her breath, she asked permission to get other nurses to come and see this funny sight.

"Sure. Why not?"

What a great start to my new medical phase!

Oh, do you want to know what inside me was connected to those wires? It didn't take too long to figure out that the wires were attached to the recently inserted AICD, which consisted of a pacemaker and a defibrillator.

Why were they just dangling there behind the bandage? I think the explanation had to do with the short time between the insertion of the AICD and my exit from Scripps Green Hospital. The time hadn't been right for cutting the wires.

The bigger question is, Why had I not noticed the clear tubes with their wires and needles, right there on my chest? My son thinks there were a variety of tapes and IV lines attached to me until just before I left the hospital. And from my vantage point, the bandage covered most of the cylinders. Besides, I wasn't keen on looking at all the medical paraphernalia clinging to me.

* * *

A few days later, my son and daughter-in-law came to take me to my first outpatient appointment at Scripps Green. Bruce, the physician's assistant who had kept my son informed throughout my ordeal, was the first person we saw. My opening remark was, "Bruce, you have some explaining to do!"

His eyes twinkled and his bushy mustache rose above his smile. Surgical scissors in hand, he was ready to cut the wires sprouting from the middle of my chest. Picture a stuffed animal with a tag on a plastic cord. The "T" end of the cord is inside the toy. To remove the tag, you push in on the toy and cut the cord. You push in so there will be no prickly plastic cord sticking out of the toy.

Well . . . Bruce was trying to be gentle, but he pushed pretty hard on my chest before cutting the wires. While I have plenty of easily pressed fatty places on my body that would not have resisted the pushing, there was no fatty "give" to the space between my breasts. Ow!

Bruce did a good job, leaving no prickly wire tips sticking out of my body. That was definitely one of our weirder interactions.

As Bruce turned away, I teased, "I don't suppose you would let me have the cylinders, would you?" Without giving me an answer, Bruce started to look through the drawers in front of him. He turned around and handed me a Ziplock bag.

Yes, inside the container were the two cylinders with purple caps. The orange and white wires with the metal "needle" tips were in the tubes, just as the nurse and I had seen them my first evening at the rehabilitation center.

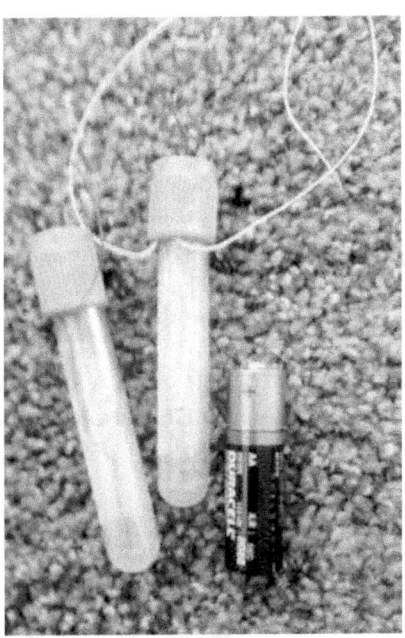

The cylinders, as compared to a AA battery

* * *

Part of my rehabilitation challenge was to assume responsibility for writing my own notes. It was time for Craig to get at least a partial break from writing all the medical notes, in addition to taking dictation from me about all my activities, thoughts, and feelings. He even managed to get in some surfing one day. Later, he took Grace to her first movie in a theater.

"Grandma, it was like a big TV, very loud, with a very long story," she told me. "I wasn't scared!"

* * *

We started right off with physical, occupational, recreational, and speech (Ha!) therapy. Back in April I'd had little use of my hands. On June 8th, I was "playing" with coins. Eyes closed, I was to find the penny among the four coins in my left hand and the two coins in my right hand, and then place it on the table. Manipulating my fingers was not easy.

The physical therapist said his job was to help me increase my stamina and overall physical condition and get me off the oxygen! It seems patients often have a hard time letting go of "needing oxygen" emotionally, if not physically.

My early occupational therapy included washing myself and brushing my teeth at the sink. Dressing myself was a slow process. The biggest thrill came when I could put on my bra by myself. Complete exhaustion followed!

The speech therapy felt more like mental testing, and made me nervous. Recreational therapy included playing poker and rummy with other patients. Decorating a ceramic trivet with colorful glass pieces was an enjoyable activity to restore small muscle control.

I did a lot of walking and stretching, stair climbing, and ball tossing. I was excited to tell Craig on the evening of June 10th that I had been off oxygen since 1:00pm. I had a feeling of satisfaction that I was doing my best.

I have a less happy, but funny, memory of a nurse running after me while I was doing my walking. She caught up with me and handed me my huge potassium pills. I was sure that after all my gains in recovery, I would die choking on a potassium pill.

The staff members were pleasant and encouraging. Then there was Vern, the singing and dancing nurse. Music always raises my spirits! One day when Craig's family was visiting me in the patio Vern came by, singing "You Are My Sunshine." Of course, I joined in. When Craig pulled out the video camera, Vern and I started doing the "Chicken Dance." Tori's eyes got sooo big!

That visit began with a surprise for my granddaughters. I was already on the patio when they arrived. As they got closer, I stood up. Grace called out, "Look, Grandma can walk!" She ran up to me, announcing that she had brought show-and-tell items in her backpack. We all had fun with the toys she shared.

✳ ✳ ✳

During my June 14th appointment with Nurse Practitioner Omana at Scripps Green Hospital Outpatient Clinic, I spoke of my queasiness, which was increasing daily. I was really hungry, but couldn't tolerate seeing or eating food. She said we could change some of my meds. She felt I needed some high-calorie liquids in addition to water. At her suggestion, we went straight to the hospital cafeteria. A fancy, calorie-dense chocolate drink was effective, fast-working "medicine." When my daughter-in-law witnessed my attitude adjustment and boost in energy after ingesting that drink, she wasted no time in heading to the store and returning with a case of Frappuccino! (I later considered listing the cost of that "medical" miracle as a tax deduction.)

I felt good. Craig took me to the ICU for a visit. The nurses who had worked so hard to keep me alive and emotionally well were overjoyed to see me smiling broadly!

✳ ✳ ✳

It was a new experience for me to have another patient in my room. Up until now I had acted as if I were the center of the universe. It's hard for me to believe I was not always polite or thinking about the feelings and needs of the people around me. Maybe my medical team did not jump the instant I called, but they did what they could for me. When you are not well, it is easy to believe "everything is all about me."

I was getting better, able to leave my room for activities. I had many visitors, telephone calls, and beautiful flowers from friends and family. Patients in ICU rooms are not allowed to receive flowers. Adding the sight and sound of friends and the beauty of flowers did wonders for me. Life was looking better every day.

My closest family-like friends, Ron and Vicki, were finally with me in person. Jason, their son, had visited me at Scripps, once I was out of the ICU. They had had to drive a long distance, and their visit meant more to me than they could possibly know. Through the years we had given each other support during several challenging events.

One of my funniest visit memories is of the evening my nephew, Jeff, popped into my room with his college-aged daughter, Ari. I was about to watch "Sex and the City" on TV. They told me to continue watching. I was way too embarrassed to watch the delightful adult-fun show, especially at the age of sixty-three, while my nephew and great niece looked on! My libido was intact, but my blushing genes took over.

* * *

On June 16th, Craig took me to an appointment with Dr. Schneider, my plastic surgeon. Instead of sending a nurse to meet me in the waiting room, the doctor came out. I was so excited to see him that I jumped (really) out of the wheelchair and walked about fifteen feet to get a hug. He was tickled by my exuberance. I, not surprisingly, ended up drained of all energy, but happy.

The doctor was pleased with the closing of the deep wound on my right leg. I still had a large indented scar that looked like a tight band around my thigh. There was a smaller scar behind my knee. He felt that neither would require plastic surgery. "I guess this will not be my first bikini year," I commented.

Trust me, I never had a body suited for a bikini.

The next day, Craig and I sat with my rehabilitation team. We heard the fabulous news that I was progressing well enough to leave in two days. I was told I could continue my recovery at Craig's home with the help of a visiting nurse. Yippee!

I have no idea what was going through Craig's mind. At least there would be fewer medical trips to see me, but having me in his home would mean more inconvenience and responsibility. I'd never had to experience what my son was handling with such grace, humor, and compassion.

To add to my excitement, I learned that Kristin and one-year-old Aengus would arrive the day after I settled in at Craig's home. Wonderful for me, but ... oh, goodie, two more people for Craig's family to accommodate. It would be like one big slumber party while two adults went to work and three little kids, all under the age of four, played around their not-too-strong grandma. Kristin was to be the chef and child watcher, especially near the long, gated flight of stairs.

My exit story is about the heist we pulled off with the help of a nurse on June 19th. I was not totally weaned off oxygen, a tank of which was to be delivered to Craig's home the next day. To alleviate my fear of needing oxygen during my first night away from a medical facility, Craig and the nurse snuck a tank of oxygen out a side door and into Craig's car. I'd like to say I was the getaway driver. Instead I sat, quietly relieved, as the two compassionate accomplices did their sneaky deed. Needless to say, the tank was returned in a timely fashion. The getaway caper was a success.

I hadn't spent a long time with the staff at Sharp Rehabilitation Center, but in twelve days I had grown fond of the people I'd met. Little did I know what an important part the Sharp Memorial Hospital system was to play in my medical future.

11

Craig's Home: Adjusting to the Outside

Mixed emotions swirled within me as Craig and I sat in the car heading to his home on June 19th. Soon I would be in a home setting with my son's family. That sounded so exciting, and so healthy. My doctors wouldn't have let me go if they didn't think I was ready. Surely now I was going in just one direction—straight ahead to full recovery. No more setbacks.

My first jolt came as we charged up the short but steep dirt path to the grassy area at the level of Craig's front door. I would have had to climb a long flight of stairs had we parked in the regular parking space.

With the help of my son and a walker, I crossed the uneven grass. By the time I was in the house, I was thrilled but totally depleted of energy. Two charming little girls to entertain me was just what I needed.

The goal now was continued improvement outside of a medical facility. I was to exercise inside, do better at eating, limit fluids, and get off the oxygen. My potassium level, weight, and blood pressure were to be monitored by a visiting nurse who would come three days a week. We learned how to change the leg bandage and keep the PICC line[1] clean.

The next afternoon I heard Kristin saying "Mommy!" in her silly "little girl" voice that always makes me laugh. There was my daughter, holding her little boy, who was now a year old. They had arrived for their two-week visit. My memory holds an idyllic image: I was happy and optimistic, surrounded by my favorite people.

My daughter-in-law made me feel at home. She helped me feel comfortable as she guided me through some of my personal care. Kristin's gift was to prepare the meals. The sad thing is that I was too listless and edgy to show them the appreciation they deserved.

I had always enjoyed anything Kristin cooked, but now my medi-

---

[1] PICC or PIC line, a peripherally inserted central catheter, is a form of intravenous access that can be used for a prolonged period of time.

cines left a metallic taste in my mouth. I ate very little yet felt overstuffed. I wanted to play with the children, but I just sat and watched.

I had my first real margarita when several relatives arrived. I imagine they were most interested in seeing Kristin and Aengus, but they each spent some time with me too.

It was the margarita that helped me feel like a real person again. Of course, my margarita had very little alcohol and just a few grains of salt on the edge of the glass.

Kristin took me to some appointments. We learned about the cardiac rehabilitation I would begin before long. We were told to watch for swelling, especially in the ankles. My weight was steadily rising, and I was experiencing loss of appetite and a bloated feeling.

* * *

Then on July 1st, just before Kristin and Aengus returned home, my primary care physician sent me back to the hospital. Recent test results had shown blood in my urine and elevated liver enzymes, and she wanted a full CT scan of my abdomen and pancreas. The hospital doctors thought she had overreacted. With my history, can you blame her?

My diuretics were adjusted, and I was released on the 4th of July with orders to stay on the oxygen, walk, and get up slowly.

By the 12th, I was dealing with more weight and "fat feet." I soon realized I needed help pulling on compression T.E.D. stockings. The tightness of the stockings forces fluid from outer tissues out into the general circulatory system so it can be peed out. I was to minimize stagnant sitting, do as much physical activity as I could tolerate, and elevate my feet above my heart as often as possible.

Craig and Grace helped the home nurse clean my intravenous wires and change the leg bandage. Grace took her work seriously. As for two-and-a-half-year-old Tori, she was caught using my long oxygen pipeline as a tightrope wire. I had to stifle my laugh as I told her to try a different gymnastic routine. Years later, both girls would enjoy attending gymnastics classes, and I would be able to watch them without worrying about my breathing.

By the 19th, my weight gain and fluid retention had led to trying a new diuretic and calling Nurse Practitioner Omana daily. Craig had prepared a chart showing the relationship between high blood pressure and my weight. "We have to get the fluid off. The weight will go with it," he insisted.

On the 22nd, by which date I weighed more and was even puffier, Dr. Rubenson approved the trial of what I began to call "my doozie diuretic." I could take two and a half milligrams of the powerful diuretic every other day in addition to my regular diuretic. On the days I added the booster, I was also to take potassium pills.

The day after my first dose of the doozie diuretic I lost eleven pounds in twenty-four hours. Boy, did I feel better! Although they told me that kidney function could be damaged by too much use of diuretics, I was happy to have the relief. I did not foresee my continuing battle with keeping my fluid levels down while preserving the health of the rest of my body.

* * *

My nephew Jeff, a San Francisco police officer, was taking some police classes in San Diego. He was able to visit me several times during the summer. Jeff's visits always perked me up.

In late July I was pleased to see Judy and Rae, two close friends from college. They were at the house when Craig and I returned from the medical appointment where I received my first dose of the doozie diuretic. I barely said hello as I ran past them to get to the bathroom. (We had already made one pit stop on the return from the doctor's office.)

It was during that visit that Judy reminded me that we had walked all over the Wild Animal Park exactly one week before my lifesaving stress treadmill test. I had been a walking time bomb!

* * *

After Kristin left, I began to experience a new wrinkle on my health journey. I was aware of a slight pain in my left breast. Poking around, I became alarmed. I tried to describe what I felt to Kristin over the phone. With my thumb and middle finger I could surround a large lump. I felt a lump shaped like a velvet-covered ring box. It felt solid and large.

Trying to imagine what I was describing, Kristin came up with a name for my mysterious intruder. From then on, we all referred to it as my "boob cube."

We tried not to worry about it. The first theory was that it was a cyst. They said it was good that it was not attached to any tissue. They told us to leave it alone.

The mammogram results looked fine. However, they scheduled me to have a sonogram the first week of August and warned me that a biopsy might be necessary.

The time when Craig's family was due to leave for Singapore was quickly approaching. They had made the decision to go a year before I became ill, and their departure date had been moved back a couple of times. August 23rd was the final target date that should not be changed.

Their dilemma was, "What do we do with Mom when we leave? It doesn't look like she will be ready to live by herself. There are still medical issues that are not neatly tied up."

This is the time to give big credit where it is due. Both Craig and his wife work at Hewlett-Packard. Craig's boss had gone out of his way to be supportive and flexible from the beginning of my health challenge, making it possible for Craig to be with me and still more or less keep up with his engineering work.

Back in April, at the start of my ICU stay, the business trip had seemed far off. As my complications piled up, Craig, my doctors, and Kristin had tried to outguess the future and think of all possible options for my care.

As is Craig's style, he kept me from being aware of the mental struggle going on. Years later, I would learn that they had wondered whether some of my close friends might let me stay with them until I could return home. Kristin wanted me to be with her in Michigan, but how could I be so far away from my doctors?

＊ ＊ ＊

In a time when we hardly ever hear good words about insurance companies, I have a rave review for Blue Shield. While I was still in the hospital, Peggy, a Blue Shield case worker, had connected with Craig. She was amazing on so many levels. She began to check on the feasibility of my going to Michigan.

I don't know that we could have pulled off this miracle if my son-in-law hadn't been doing his post-doctoral work at the University of Michigan. The university has a large and famous hospital. My Blue Shield policy allowed me to transfer my benefits to Ann Arbor as long as I stayed there at least three months. They set me up with a full slate of doctors, a lab, and a cardiac rehabilitation center.

Peggy and Diane, another Blue Shield staff member, did the research and paperwork to make my transfer possible. They were enormously pleasant and helpful to Craig.

At one point Craig came into my room and said, "I have been looking at the expense statements from Blue Shield. I haven't written anything down, but I believe your medical expenses have exceeded a million dollars."

Yes, I'd had medical insurance deductions taken out of my teacher's paycheck for many years, but that money could not come close to paying my recent bills. I worry about people who don't have insurance. It may seem a big expense, but being without insurance is way too big a gamble.

✶ ✶ ✶

I was to fly to Kristin's home on August 12th. Based on my last appointments, we had several issues to address:

- A staph infection that had reappeared on my leg and was being treated with an IV medication while I was at Craig's house. I needed to switch to an oral antibiotic.
- Getting a sonogram of the "boob cube."
- Picking up my medical records and San Diego doctors' notes to take to my Michigan doctors.

The day arrived for the sonogram of my "boob cube." Yea! No sign of cancer! The lump was non-calcified. It might need to be cut out later, but it would probably dissolve on its own. The term for it is "fat necrosis," a condition caused by trauma or infection in which neutral tissue fats are broken down into fatty acids and glycerol. Fat necrosis occurs most commonly in the breasts and subcutaneous areas.

With the worry about the "boob cube" out of the way, I was emotionally ready to leave California.

✶ ✶ ✶

My first night in my own home since March 29th was the night before I flew to Michigan. Trying to pack for a three-month stay at my daughter's home, I was overwhelmed with decisions. My low energy turned the physical activity of packing into a real challenge, testing my nerves and sanity.

My son arrived early the next morning, but later than he'd planned. All I remember is a flurry of arms stuffing clothes and other paraphernalia into suitcases. Then came the mighty labor to get the zippers shut. "Oh, don't forget my walker."

Thank goodness, we didn't have to handle an oxygen tank. The airline had its own setup.

At the airport there was more fussing with the suitcases. We had to redistribute the weight from one suitcase to another—yes, right there on the floor in front of the counter.

After a hurried but warm goodbye hug with Craig, it was finally time for the airport staff to whisk me away. Due to my pacemaker/defibrillator, security officers gave me a pat-down tickle test.

Was it time for Craig to heave a huge sigh of relief? His "mother shift" had come to an end. Of course, now it was time to zoom into top speed to get his family ready to leave for their year in Singapore. My dearest hope was that he could get a breather before their departure. He deserved time alone with his wife and daughters.

12

Kristin's Home in Michigan: Developing Independence

Kristin met me at the Detroit airport late on August 12th. We had no trouble finding my suitcases. Thank goodness, they had not split open. My daughter saw a walker on the luggage carousel, but I said it couldn't be mine because mine was black, not purple.

Seeing it coming around for the third time, she decided to check the tag. Yep, it had my name on it. It seems the bright airport lights showed the true color of the Stingray, my hotshot purple walking aid!

The next bit of trauma involved opening my big suitcase. It had come with a combination lock I had not bothered to learn how to use. So that suitcases could be inspected at the airport, we had been told not to use our locks. When I tried to open my suitcase in my new sleeping quarters, I discovered that it had somehow contrived to lock itself.

My son-in-law Brian and his friend spent a long time trying to guess the lock combination. They were sure they could break the code and avoid having to cut my suitcase open. I was afraid my suitcase would burst open at some point, and after they broke the code, it did! With much embarrassment I told them to turn away. I didn't want them to see my huge "grannie panties"! (For comfort during my blocked-fluid days, I had purchased oversized underwear.)

✶ ✶ ✶

The goal for this part of my recovery was continued physical improvement while becoming independent and able to care for myself. As I met my new doctors, I was happy to have Kristin as my patient advocate. Her presence helped me transition to my new medical team, and her encouragement helped me believe I was capable of taking care of myself. She was always a cell-phone call away if I needed extra help.

On August 20th, Peggy called from Blue Shield to see how the transition was going. I was happy to give her a good report.

We looked into assistance for transportation to medical appointments. The most helpful plan would not be available to me until a week before I returned to California. In the interim, I got used to walking the few blocks to the closest bus stop with my walker.

I was used to being the driver. I learned how complicated it can be for people who don't drive and/or have disabilities. I met helpful bystanders and bus drivers, but I also encountered rude or impatient people. Thank goodness I always dealt with public transportation during the day. I never felt afraid. I also had plenty of time to figure out how to get where I needed to go.

✳ ✳ ✳

In Michigan, while the fluid was a continuing concern, my need for oxygen had decreased. By mid-October, I was able to call the healthcare company to tell them to take the big, noisy oxygen setup away.

My cardiac rehabilitation began in early October. I went three times a week. The atmosphere was informal, and I soon felt like a club member. The room with the exercise equipment was not big.

I would peddle my bike, far from the desk with the monitoring screen, until I heard the shout-out, "Linda, slow down. Your pulse is too high."

My heart had taken quite a beating, so my progress was slow, but steady. I enjoyed the camaraderie, the stories from other patients, and the Beach Boys music they often played for the "California girl."

One day I arrived an hour early, having forgotten that we were to start later that day. My mistake led to a wonderful talk with a World War II veteran who had also forgotten about our time change. My dad had been in the Pacific during World War II, and I had lots of questions that brought out many detailed stories. I asked my friend whether he had told these stories to his family. Like many veterans, he did not share his horrible memories until Tom Brokaw published his book, *The Greatest Generation*, in 1998.

As so often happens, our missteps lead us to new treasures. Arriving at the wrong time had brought a super reward!

✳ ✳ ✳

While chatting with other patients, I heard what happened if your internal defibrillator "went off." Internal defibrillators (ICD/AICD) are implanted in the body. Like external portable defibrillators, they work by inducing a shock to the heart that corrects a potentially fatal heart arrhythmia. A person with an internal defibrillator may not be able to feel an arrhythmia, but when it is corrected by the ICD they feel the shock that has been delivered. My AICD combined the defibrillator with a pacemaker.

I don't remember being told at the hospital about the strong kickback a person might experience. The man on the exercise bike next to mine described an experience he'd had while putting groceries into the trunk of his car. Boom! He'd found himself thrust backward some three to five feet when his ICD went into action.

I vowed then and there that I would never need the use of my defibrillator!

The time had come to try Coumadin (Warfarin) again. This blood thinner (anticoagulant) helps to prevent new blood clots from forming and to keep existing blood clots from getting worse. My Scripps Green doctors had tried to start me on it, but my body couldn't handle it at that time.

This medicine was serious blood-thinning stuff. A small cut on the finger could become a bloody mess. Due to my prior bleeding problems, they watched me carefully after I took my first dose. Later that day, Kristin teased me about using knives. "That's okay, Mom, I'll chop the carrots." I did tolerate the medicine, but I now had to have more frequent lab visits in Ann Arbor and after I returned to California.

Accustomed to driving my own car, I was not looking forward to commuting with the inflexibility of using public transportation to get to the cardiac rehab facility three times a week. I will now confess to a plan I devised on my own in early October, without anybody's approval.

Becoming independent was a big goal, right?

Kristin and Brian had left with Aengus and one of the dogs for a three-day vacation, leaving me in the company of the other dog. A neighbor had agreed to look in on me. I made my move a few days before the start of my cardiac rehabilitation program: I rented a bright-red car!

Many years earlier I had heard, "It is easier to ask forgiveness than to beg for permission." My daughter could understand why I believed I needed a car, but she was not pleased that I had chosen to act without checking with my doctors or the family.

Having that car made life decidedly easier for me. Not only could I get to my many appointments, I could also get out of the house for my own amusement. In addition, I was also able to give Kristin's family more alone time in the evenings and during weekends.

One day Kristin had taken me to a massage salon that offered fifteen-minute chair massages. Once I rented the car, I could get more massages. Adding massage for my head, feet, and legs just about had me purring. On other occasions I got a manicure and pedicure, participated in singing and dancing for peace ("Sufi Dancing"), ate at an Indian restaurant, went to a comedy club, and enjoyed a long Sunday drive—all by myself.

* * *

I had a truly special treat when my longtime friend Arvind visited me from his home in Indianapolis. We had met as pen pals when we were both in high school, he in Bombay (now Mumbai) and I in Monrovia, California. Later, he earned graduate degrees in the United States and chose to stay here. Our friendship had continued.

Rather than go to a restaurant, we accepted Kristin's offer to cook for us. I'm pleased that Arvind and Kristin had a chance to get to know each other better. Of course, my grandson, Aengus, provided the entertainment.

* * *

Kristin had disrupted their office space to set up a downstairs bedroom for me. You should have seen the candy stash I hoarded on the shelves to one side of my bed! I had tried to limit sweets, especially candy, for years. Now that I was on a serious restriction diet, low in fat, salt, and fluids, I decided that a small amount of candy could be allowed. Peppermint patties were the star attraction.

We all worried that the dogs might swallow some of my pills. I was taking a lot of strong medicine at the time. I did my best to handle my medicine carefully and not let any pills sneak away from me. We made it through the three and a half months without a catastrophe. Whew!

I had a nice social life in Ann Arbor. During my first month there, I ate at Conner O'Neil's (an Irish pub), feasted on Zingerman's outstanding bread, and enjoyed visits with family friends and the fancy breakfasts Kristin prepared. My appetite had improved. We attended a University of Michigan Science Department picnic where kids, dogs, and grandmas were welcome. I was decidedly not living in a medical facility anymore!

Kristin introduced me to friends of hers who began to take me out for lunch, movies, and shopping. Pat and Lottie did a great job of helping me feel I was not just a patient. This transition phase worked better than we could have anticipated. Had I gone to my own home, I'm sure I would have been too afraid to leave my condo.

The fall leaves were beginning to arrive. In southern California, only a few token trees have foliage that changes color. It makes it tough to help our young children understand the term "seasons." In Michigan, I would look down the street daily for signs of the big change. Being sick afforded me the opportunity to view the magical, show-stopping turning of the leaves in the midwestern section of our country.

Kristin, Aengus, and I went for a drive through the glorious landscape. I had not been warned that we would drive to Hell and back. In Michigan there is a small town named Hell, where there is a year-round Halloween-inspired store. It was fun watching my seventeen-month-old grandson take in the scary ghosts, goblins, witches—anything bloody. He was captivated by a "body" that would suddenly drop, leaving its head behind. He was young enough to enjoy the action while not being aware of the scary aspect.

✳ ✳ ✳

I had the fun of observing curious Aengus scooting around, exploring nooks and crannies while making up his own games. Here comes my favorite story: Early one evening, Brian showed Aengus how dogs shake hands. "How do you do?" Brian asked one dog. At that point, up would come a paw and the handshake would take place. Aengus watched with interest.

Then Brian asked Aengus, "How do you do?" He reached for Aengus's hand to shake it. Aengus looked perplexed. Brian tried again, asking, "How do you do?" while reaching for my grandson's hand. This time Aengus pulled back his hand and lifted his foot to touch Brian's hand. I thought I would bust a gut. I laughed as silently as possible! Dogs don't have hands, silly Daddy.

The combination of observing that priceless gem and then being startled and worried when Aengus climbed a stepladder in the kitchen to reach a high shelf loosened my funny bone and released my self-centered-ness. I became more aware of what was happening around me. My protective mothering instincts were returning.

I was recovering, on so many levels.

My favorite thrill was seeing Aengus run down the hall to my bedroom after he and Kristin arrived home from daycare and work one evening. My grandson called out, "Yamma! Yamma!" Interestingly, within a few days he changed Yamma to Yamai (pronounced like Hawaii). That is the name that stuck for me and for his other grandmother. I love my special name!

Meanwhile, we received telephone calls from Craig's family in Singapore. They were having wonderful adventures. Both girls attended a preschool in the mall connected to their building. Grace told me all about her four-year-old birthday celebration in the Kids' Lounge of the high-rise apartment building.

In Ann Arbor I got in on the traditional carving of jack-o-lanterns, a visit from Brian's mother, and a University of Michigan hockey game. Having attended a small college, I found the contrast of witnessing activities connected to a huge Homecoming football game impressive. I watched alumni and current band members rehearsing for halftime and was wowed by the drum-line routine. My long walk home after a private celebration party just about did me in, but my spirit was riding high! Did I see the football game? No, but we heard the announcer's play-by-play in our backyard.

Before returning to California, I held the newest cousin and attended a wedding. We changed my November 12th airline ticket to December 4th so I could be with Brian's family for Thanksgiving. They had a craft table set up for decorating Christmas tree ornaments. To commemorate my most unusual year, I wrote 2004 on mine. I do make sure it goes up on my tree every year.

Kristin had done well with her stewardship of my "becoming independent" phase. She had introduced me to people who treated me like a normal person, not a sick person, and encouraged me to take on activities that fired up a new feeling of vitality. When I talked too much about my pills or diet, she had given me positive suggestions I could follow. I was beginning to believe in my ability to care for myself.

She has continued to be my most supportive fan, recognizing how much I have changed, especially as I developed self-confidence. As new dips on the roller coaster presented themselves, she allowed me to express my feelings and then reminded me about the storms I had weathered. She let me cry until I was ready to laugh at myself.

✷ ✷ ✷

A sign that we had achieved my medical and emotional goals came when I realized I was finally ready to go home to Carlsbad. I was no longer afraid to live alone.

In preparation for my return home, I needed to reinstate my California doctors, set up my first appointments, receive a "Certificate of Participation" from the Cardiac Rehabilitation Center in Ann Arbor, and start packing.

By the way, I'm sure I "graduated" at the bottom of my rehab class. I still had a lot of improving to do.

✷ ✷ ✷

We must have packed a box or two to mail. I had bought several items of cold weather clothing and gathered a few souvenirs during my visit. New friends had told me about two really nice thrift shops where the proceeds went to schools and women's projects. I hardly ever get a chance to wear my long red flannel house gown with the big snowman on it. We seldom get those super-cold-hot-chocolate-cuddle-up-by-the-fire days in my town.

I did carry onto the plane an eighteen-inch-high plush snow lady carrying her snow baby. To this day, when I put away my December decorations I put out snowflakes and snowmen made from a variety of materials. They are often on display until late spring, since other parts of our country may still have real snow while we bask in bright sunlight in Carlsbad.

13

Back Home at Last!

My flight home on December 4th was uneventful. That's good, because I am not an enthusiastic airline passenger. Nevertheless, I usually enjoy meeting people in the airport and on the plane.

I was supposed to be picked up at the airport by my daughter-in-law's sister. At the last minute her plans changed, leaving her husband with the task. I was a bit embarrassed to tell him I wanted to sit in the back seat with my two suitcases. I had to explain that I couldn't remember what I had done with the key to my front door. I don't recall where I eventually found it. I just know that I couldn't find it in my purse or in my carry-on bag. What a relief that we did not have to bash down my front door!

There I was, at home to stay, eight months after my treadmill stress test. Craig's family was nearly ten thousand miles away, and I had just one close friend in the area. I wondered whether I would ever have even a small group of close friends. While I had met nice people at the senior center and the library, and the people living on my cul-de-sac were friendly, they were not yet close friends. We had put on a few block parties together. I felt closest to my next-door neighbors. Their primary home was in Florida, so I didn't get to visit with them often.

Lying in my own bed, feeling much healthier than when I'd left Carlsbad in August, I eased into a good night's sleep.

Sunday, December 5th, was my first full day at home. Jason, whom I often refer to as my pretend nephew, came over that morning from the University of California, San Diego, to help check out my car after its long period of disuse. I also had him carry in many boxes of holiday decorations from my garage so I could slowly jolly-up my home.

While I was in the garage by myself, a woman looked in as she walked past. JoAnn had just moved into our complex. She'd retired a bit early and moved to San Diego to be here in time for the birth of her grandchild.

We clicked immediately. We had both been teachers, though she had moved further up the ranks than I. She'd moved here to be with her daughter, who was expecting a baby any day. Both of us had looked forward to being hands-on grandmothers from Day One.

I had no idea at the time that JoAnn and I would form a deep and supportive bond. I had had a few good and true friends through the years, but never one who lived only a few doors away.

I'm sure JoAnn could write the rest of this book. Though I was by no means her main concern, she saw what was happening to me and talked with me about the changes I was experiencing. She saw past my outward persona and upbeat personality, and was gentle with me during my not-so-pleasant days.

✶ ✶ ✶

December 6th was the first time I went to a Scripps Green Hospital Outpatient Clinic appointment without my son pushing me in a wheelchair through the maze of hallways. I was on my own, with no wheelchair or walker.

Nurse Practitioner Omana didn't make any changes to my meds or self-care except to set me up with the Coumadin (Warfarin) Clinic close to my home. I went weekly to have a blood test to see how long it took my blood to clot.

The other concern, of course, was fluid buildup. I was told to keep a daily record of my morning weight, as rapidly increasing weight would indicate fluid accumulation in my body.

One of the goals of the clinic is to help patients learn self-management skills that will help to keep them from returning to the hospital.

My medical team had taught me about my heart condition and the medicines I needed to take. My responsibility now was to incorporate new health habits and find activities that bolstered my spirit. I took seriously the information I'd learned from the "Healthy Living" lectures in Ann Arbor.

I went to the library and bookstores to find cookbooks that dealt with heart disease. The best and worst one I bought was called *The No Salt, Lowest-Sodium Cookbook*. Before my sister came for our Christmas celebration, I tested some recipes. Yuck! In deference to the author, the suggestions were good, considering the constraints.

I had a lot to learn about how to handle my condition.

Then I got a book that included recipes meant to duplicate famous dishes from around the world. The recipe names and backstories were inviting, but the medicines I was taking must have interfered with my taste buds. Only recipes with very few ingredients were edible. Lemon juice helped, but the carefully chosen herbs did not awaken any desire in me. I had no interest in fussing with fresh herbs, and my spices were probably way too old.

I decided I preferred eating the individual main ingredients without following long recipes. Instead of preparing a low-salt, low-fat, low-sugar version of Green Beans Almandine, I would heat the beans and drizzle them with lemon juice, and then alternate bites of beans with bites of almonds.

I had learned in the heart-healthy cooking lectures that apple cider vinegar, yellow mustard, and horseradish are good additions to lemon juice for waking up the taste buds.

* * *

My sister Marilyn and I had both had health scares in 2004. It was time to be grateful for the family members and friends who supported us and had put their lives on hold to help us survive. It was also time for us to celebrate (albeit very carefully) what we had done to help ourselves get better.

Marilyn was coming to visit, and I was determined to make this holiday season enjoyable and a bit unique for us. Recent Christmas fun had involved family, kids, dogs, singing carols, lots of presents under the tree, and holiday food in bigger quantities than at other times of the year. What could we do this season to "give back" or "pay forward" the help we had been given? Was it too late to sign up to deliver gifts or food to needy families?

I called the Carlsbad City Hall to see whether someone there could connect us with an organization that could use our help. Sue, the city's Community Coordinator, had no projects at the time, but she encouraged me to sign up to volunteer at a later date. She did suggest contacting Brother Benno's. Their mission: to distribute the generous gifts entrusted to them by the community, and to serve and uplift the dignity of those in dire need in north-coastal San Diego County.

I was pleased to learn that my sister and I would be able to help in the "Gift-Giving Shop," where we would offer towels, toiletries, clothes, toys, and more on Christmas morning. "Guests" would then go into the dining room for a delicious holiday dinner with all the trimmings. (I love the fact that the Foundation chooses to refer to the people they serve as guests.)

Marilyn arrived and the atmosphere in my home got lighter. Holiday calls and cards from Kristin's family and out-of-town friends and relatives raised our spirits. We decorated my artificial tree a little at a time. We vowed that we would sing our favorite carols on Christmas Eve, even if we were the only ones in the house.

We enjoyed the special treat of going to the home of my daughter-in-law's parents. They had a web camera connected to their computer, which we turned on at an agreed-upon time. There must have been at least twelve excited family members calling out and waving to Craig's family—in their Singapore apartment! They looked so happy. Our best Christmas present that year was seeing them enjoying their well-deserved, exciting adventure so far away.

Our very different Christmas morning began slowly, without the usual fun of getting ready to go to my son's home. No precious little girls to watch as they unwrapped and played with new toys. I don't remember whether I felt moments of melancholy over that.

Excitement began to grow as we arrived at the Brother Benno's site. People in Santa hats and colorful clothes bustled around in preparation to receive the first guests. I was soon immersed in compassionate good feeling in a room stacked with useful and nonessential treats. I was tired when our shift was over, but didn't want to leave.

We chose to share our holiday meal at a restaurant near Brother Benno's where we saw a few other volunteers. The meal may have been nondescript, but the way we celebrated Christmas was special.

Later, we had pizza and a small glass of wine at home. I sent off emails to my son and daughter, wishing them Merry Christmas. I said we had found a way to bring joy to others and ourselves at the end of what had been for us a most unusual year. I must have mentioned the pizza and wine, because I received understandably negative comments from my kids. "Pizza? With all its fat and salt? Wine? How much wine?"

I replied that I had prepared a ridiculously bland pizza from a recipe in one of my heart-healthy cookbooks. As unappealing as it was, we had eaten a very small amount. The apple-and-nuts side dish had tasted far better. The wine had been in a little plastic bottle we shared, so we couldn't have had much.

Before and after preparing the pizza, I tried out several other recipes. My sister was the main guinea-pig taster. She is a kind soul, easy to please. As she took a bite of each new concoction and smiled her approval, I stood next to my food disposal system. If my first bites made me cringe, I simply scraped the culinary "delight" into the grinding hole. With weird glee, I flipped the switch. Gone!

Early on New Year's Eve day we got a funny, yet serious, call from Singapore. Craig said they were already in the new year, 2005. Yea! 2004 was over for them. Soon it would be over for us, too.

Marilyn and I shared a Happy New Year hug at midnight. I couldn't help wondering what was in store in 2005.

14

Taking Charge in 2005

My sole purpose in 2005 was to move forward on my heart journey. I was determined not to let down my family and friends or the nurses and doctors who had guided, encouraged, and dragged me through the turbulence I had faced in 2004.

My son's family was in Singapore, my daughter's family was in Michigan, and my sister and nephew were in the San Francisco Bay Area. As the baby in my birth family, I may have relied on that role a bit too much as I was growing up. My severe illness had perhaps moved me backward on the maturity scale. It was time to see what strength and courage I could muster.

This was the time for drawing strength from my Finnish background. All four of my grandparents were born in Finland. I had visited relatives on both sides of my family there, and had developed strong bonds in recent years with members of my father's side of the family. I'd grown up with the last name Savolaine, not-at-all Finnish sounding. I had learned long ago that the original final 'n' had been removed when my immigrant grandfather came through Ellis Island in 1900.

In 2005, I wanted to claim the power of *sisu* that comes with my true last name: *Savolainen*. (*Sisu* is a Finnish word referring to determination, bravery, and resilience. However, the word is widely considered to lack a proper translation into any other language. According to Wikipedia.org, "*Sisu* is about taking action against the odds and displaying courage and resoluteness in the face of adversity.")

✶ ✶ ✶

It was time to go back to my gym. The personal trainer I'd worked with before was not available, so I was introduced to Joel, another trainer. Having taken extra classes and received many certifications in rehabilitation, Joel convinced me he would be able to help me. Indeed, as my heart condition worsened, Joel knew just what exercises, compassionate words, and hugs would suit me best at each fluctuation of my emotional and physical state.

∗ ∗ ∗

In keeping with a promise to myself to enhance my emotional health by getting involved in new activities and meeting new people, it was time to make good on my agreement with Sue by doing some volunteering.

Among a variety of smaller tasks, I chose to co-lead a series of lessons for third graders. My friend and I taught "City Stuff," an interesting curriculum designed to take the young students into the inner workings of the City of Carlsbad and the services it provided. Working with the class over several weeks was most enjoyable.

As for my social life, I reconnected with Marilyn A., a woman I had met at a book club. She was totally wheelchair-bound and drove her van with hand-control adaptations, since she could not use her legs. Her multiple sclerosis did not limit our fun together. She and I went to movies and concerts, took the train to San Diego, watched TV, and worked on puzzles together. We came from vastly different backgrounds. Sharing our stories brought out big laughs as well as some tears.

I got together with condo neighbors JoAnn and Sue whenever there was an opening in our collective schedules. Email, phone calls, and infrequent visits kept me in touch with college friends as well. I also deepened my relationship with two women I'd met at an Elderhostel week in Arizona. Before I'd become ill, we had visited each other's homes.

∗ ∗ ∗

After one of my outpatient appointments at Scripps Green Hospital, I decided to visit the ICU. Would any of the nurses remember me? It was January, seven months after my long stay in 2004. I got a rousing welcome as I walked through the unit. "I danced through the ICU!" I wrote in emails to my kids. They both liked my choice of words.

∗ ∗ ∗

Omana, NP, had told me to record my morning weight each day. One day, I realized I had gained four pounds in six days while taking my twice-daily low dose of a diuretic. She told me to increase doses of my "booster diuretic" to three times a week. The morning after my "booster (doozie) pill," I often dropped two to three pounds.

All this time, I was eating light, healthy meals. As soon as I finished eating, I'd feel bloated. It's a good thing my meals were so bland. I can't imagine how I would have felt if I'd been gaining fluid weight and food weight!

My doctor added a strong beta-blocker[1] drug to my list of medicines in mid-March. I was to take just a "fairy dust" amount at first.

The side effects that came with my high-fluid days were clear and predictable. Yes, even two to four extra pounds of fluid felt physically painful. The extra weight affected my posture, causing me to bend over while walking. My energy level went down, and my raw, fragile emotions went haywire.

Most of the time I saw myself as healthy and happy with a medical challenge I could handle. But as a precaution, my doctor prescribed nitroglycerin[2] to use in case of chest pain.

On February 16th I had an afternoon cardiologist appointment and an evening echo (heart strength) appointment. Between the appointments I stayed in the cafeteria, eating dinner and reading. Just before leaving the cafeteria, I went to get a drink of water. I became excited when I caught a glimpse of a man I was almost sure was the respiratory therapist who had frequently stopped by my room in the ICU on his way to see his patients who had breathing issues. Many times he had waved and said "Hi," but later he'd added, "We have to get you up dancing!"

I situated myself in a spot where he would see me as he came around the corner. When he came into my view, I said, "Shall we dance?" He gave me a strange look. I repeated my invitation. After a long pause I became embarrassed, thinking I was talking to the wrong person. Flustered, I asked, "Do you work in the ICU?"

His face lit up and he exclaimed, "Is that you?" He had seen me only at night, lying in bed. After we laughed, talked, and hugged, we struck a dancing pose so the cashier could snap a photo with my camera. That was a true high point for me! The photo is now in my *New Heart Adventure* scrapbook.

---

[1] Beta blockers affect the heart and circulation. They are used to treat a weak heart and hypertension (high blood pressure).

[2] Nitroglycerin dilates (widens) blood vessels, making it easier for the heart to pump blood through them. It is used to treat or prevent angina, the clinical name for chest pain caused by an insufficient blood supply to the heart.

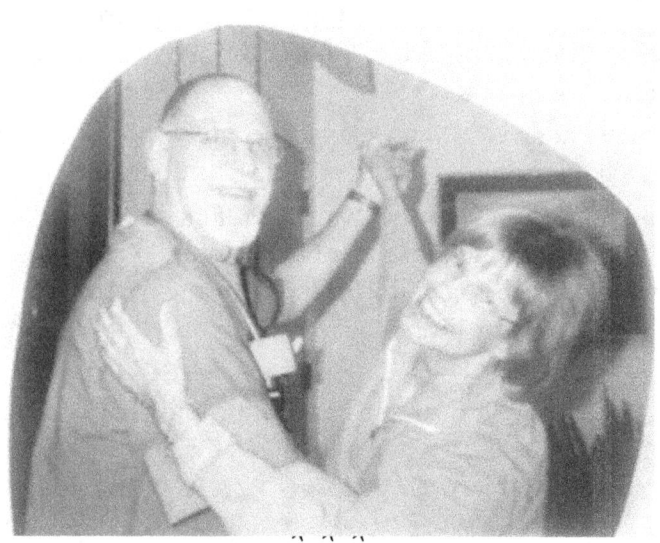

From a couple of sources I had heard about the Scripps Integrative Medicine Healing Hearts Program, an integrative medical approach for recovering patients who wanted to live a healthier life. The mind, body, and spirit were considered in this proactive series of classes. It was administered by Dr. Erminia (Mimi) Guarneri and held in the Shiley Pavilion on the Scripps Green Hospital campus.

Jim, my financial advisor, helped me enroll in the program, which he had already experienced.

While my insurance would cover my second monitored exercise program, it wouldn't cover the healthy living classes in the three-month series. When I asked Jim whether I could afford the program, he was adamant. "You can't afford not to have this experience!" he said.

I was to start the program when I returned from a special trip. My son had invited my sister and me to visit his family in Singapore. I asked my doctor whether my health could withstand the trip. He gave his unequivocal approval.

I am a bit skittish about flying. Added to my low-level fear of flying was my nervousness about being far from my doctors, even though we had reached a plateau at which the diuretics I was taking balanced out my continuing weight gain.

On the other hand, how could I possibly give up an opportunity to visit my son's family in an exotic location? The abundant telephone calls, photos, and videos couldn't take the place of face-to-face fun.

The visit brought me many highs as we enjoyed frequent sightseeing excursions, eating a wide variety of delectable international foods, and observing the hustle and bustle of people and traffic in a vibrant metropolitan setting.

My challenges consisted of trying to keep up with my family's ability to get around and missing out on activities when I felt I needed to rest. While in Singapore, I learned more about what had happened around me during my ICU stay and rehabilitation the previous year.

Hearing all the details made me feel like I was watching a play in which I was the central character. While the play was going on in 2004, I had been concerned with only my part. As I was made aware of the total story, I imagined myself in the audience, now able to see and understand more about the roles the other characters played. The more I knew, the guiltier I felt. About getting sick. About needing so much help. About my less-than-polite manner. Or . . . was I just wallowing in the attention?

✶ ✶ ✶

My most unusual souvenir was a Singapore magazine titled *Family* (much like *Parents* or *Family Circle* in our country), filled with articles about parenting. I was handed the magazine during a quiet time. As I skimmed through it, I did a double take when I saw some pictures accompanying an article about naughty behaviors of young children. There in big, colorful spreads were the priceless faces of both my granddaughters! My little actresses were displaying their versions of "Who, me?" and "Not me!" facial expressions.

I hurried into the living room. "Okay," I said, "what is the story?"

It seems the girls had been noticed in the mall on the way home from preschool with Mommy, and the family had accepted the invitation to have the girls photographed. I had the fun of taking copies of the magazine home with me, one for me and one for the other grandmother in San Diego. She received her copy on Mothers Day, 2005. How appropriate!

On the long flight home, I replayed in my mind my daughter's words from just before the trip: "Mom, it is amazing to know how well you are now, after being so seriously ill for most of last year!"

✶ ✶ ✶

May 12th was a good example of a day with emotional high and low ripples. My daughter-in-law had bought lovely presents in Singapore for the nurses and doctors who had been especially helpful when I was in Scripps Green Hospital. I had the fun of delivering the gifts after I returned home. I heard beautiful compliments about my family. I was just the messenger, but I took in the warm words and hugs from the staff members.

Then I hurried over to another site to take a treadmill stress test. We needed a baseline reading to use as a comparison for the reading to be taken at the end of the Healing Hearts program. I was looking and feeling good. Out of the blue, I became nervous and emotional when I saw the treadmill in that medical setting.

"Remember, everything has been fixed," they told me. Nevertheless, my noticeably negative flashback reaction caused the nurse to send for a doctor. Once I started chatting with the doctor—probably about my grandchildren—I was fine.

Just before I left the room, a different nurse came in. She introduced herself as the nurse who'd been on duty during my March 2004 stress treadmill test. She said, "I am the one who started this whole mess." I gave her an extra-warm hug as I thanked her for her concern and for calling in Dr. Rubenson. "You were one sick puppy," she reminded me.

I was back to good spirits the next day for my workout with my trainer after a good session on the treadmill in the gym.

✳ ✳ ✳

The day arrived for the start of the Healing Hearts program. During the intake interview, a program psychologist read off a list of stressors that could lead to heart problems:

> Death of a loved one
> Divorce
> Move to a new location
> Persecution complex
> Pessimism
> Anger
> Fear

While I had experienced all of the first three, I denied that any of them had caused me excess stress. As far as the last four were concerned, no, I was basically an upbeat person.

Then the psychologist used the phrase "repressed hostility," and I said, "Bingo!" I often felt powerless to speak up for myself or help someone else who was being ridiculed or mistreated. I had never experienced physical or emotional beatings. For the most part, I had nothing to complain about. I think I am just one of that large class of people who are extra-sensitive and feel subordinate to the confident people surrounding them.

The Healing Hearts participants met three times a week for three months, starting each day with monitored exercise. We participated in continuing sessions or lectures involving music therapy, spirituality, yoga, vegetarian cooking, meditation, Healing Touch, biofeedback, and guided imagery. I clearly remember whispering at the end of each session of yoga exercises with guided meditation, "What a gift!"

Our support group interaction affected me deeply. We talked about our medical challenges and shared stress-reduction methods we had tried. As we grew closer, we were able to express our fears and tell stories that would not be appropriate in settings with people who had not experienced similar challenges.

15
I'm 65 and I'm *Alive!*

In early May of 2005 I needed to postpone an outpatient appointment. Since I would have had to wait a long time for the next available appointment with Dr. Rubenson, I was encouraged to see a doctor who was about to join my clinic. Omana said his name was Dr. Heywood, and that I should call the scheduling department to set up the appointment. She told me he had left a practice with the well-respected Loma Linda University Hospital to move to the San Diego area. I heard that his credentials were impressive and that he had a wonderful bedside manner.

I hit a snag when I called the scheduler. After telling me that the new cardiologist worked in the Congestive Heart Failure Clinic, she asked, "Do you have congestive heart failure?"

I had never heard that scary term connected to my situation. "I don't know," I said. "I had five bypasses that hyperclotted, and I was in the ICU for nine weeks." I was becoming agitated, feeling teary. Then I said, "Wait. My nurse, Omana, said I could see him."

That was the day I learned the name for my particular heart problem. I hadn't even realized that all of my outpatient cardiac appointments since my release from Scripps Green Hospital had taken place in the Congestive Heart Failure Clinic.

Years later, Craig told me he had learned the name for my condition when he had set up my first outpatient appointment with Omana in June of 2004. His most important question for Omana had been, "Why were we told to go to the Congestive Heart Failure Clinic?" Just before we left the hospital, he'd been told by Dr. Grudko that I had an ejection fraction[1] of 35%.

---

[1] The term "ejection fraction," also known as "EF," refers to the percentage of blood pumped out of a filled ventricle with each heartbeat. The EF is the numerical result of an echocardiogram (echo).

Craig was not told that an ejection fraction of 40% or lower is one criterion used to designate a patient as having congestive heart failure.[1] No further information had been given at that time, leaving Omana with the task of filling in the blanks about my medical condition.

If Omana had answered Craig's questions while I was in the room, her explanations had gone right over my head. Maybe I hadn't been ready to acknowledge the medical details. The new doctor would have to give me answers to the same questions Craig had discussed with Omana.

On May 18th, I had my first appointment with Dr. J. Thomas Heywood, a tall man with a big smile. We got off to a good start when he gently answered my questions about this condition I now knew I had.

I learned that my ejection fraction had been 35% at the time I left the hospital. Did that mean my heart was working at just 35% of a complete 100% capacity? That sounded terrible, since I considered the EF an indication of the strength of the heart. I was comforted, to a small degree, to learn that the average EF of a healthy woman my age was 50%.

I asked my new doctor to recommend a book that would give me more information about congestive heart failure. On my way home, I bought the book he'd recommended.

I liked his manner and felt he would be a good addition to my medical team—that is, until he ended my appointment with this comment to Omana: "We can't have her taking these high doses of diuretics."

Omana darted out of the door after him, calling out, "You haven't seen what happens to her." His bedside manner didn't seem so good at that point.

Years later, when I decided to write a book, I requested hospital records and doctors' notes. On May 18th we had discussed my EF of 35%. The records below show my ejection fraction, based on the echo administered later that same day.

Excerpts from the hospital record from that first appointment include:

---

[1] Congestive heart failure is a weakness of the heart that leads to a buildup of fluid in the lungs and surrounding body tissues. With heart failure, blood moves through the heart and body at a slower rate, and pressure in the heart increases. As a result, the heart cannot pump enough oxygen and nutrients to meet the body's needs. If fluid builds up in the arms, legs, ankles, feet, lungs, or other organs, the body becomes congested.

> **Hospital Records, May 18, 2005**
>
> EF 20%
>
> She is concerned about exercising and wants to know what is the right amount.
>
> Low blood pressure readings
>
> 121 pounds
>
> I am going to stop her Zaroxolyn at this time.
>
> Alert female, looking younger than her stated age

Uh oh, my EF number was down even more. But on the up side, I loved what he'd said about my looks! My personal notes after the May 18th visit do not include the EF of 20%. I was not aware of my declining heart strength.

At my appointment with Dr. Heywood on the 26th, I told him about the Healing Hearts program. I went into my fast and happy talking with animated hand motions. I knew I was going to benefit from the stress-reducing options and the support group.

Within seconds, my doctor saw the other side of me on a high-fluid day. Out came the tears and my admission of my fears about my condition.

So what was the good doctor's prescription after seeing the true me? He decided I did indeed need regular boosts of my doozie diuretic. Thank heaven! I was becoming fond of my new doctor.

His next piece of advice cinched my admiration for his medical expertise. He agreed that I should learn and practice yoga and other calming techniques. Then he added, "You need lots of laughing."

I enjoyed reading the medical notes from that appointment years later. Here are my favorite parts:

> **Hospital Records, May 26, 2005**
>
> We attempted to decrease her diuretics because of marginal blood pressures. She did not tolerate this at all. She had a four- to five-pound weight gain and felt bad.
>
> She did take Zaroxolyn at home, lost four pounds and felt better.
>
> Her blood pressure today is better . . .
>
> She is going to the exercise class and enjoys that . . . is able to walk twenty minutes or so.

> [Go back to] Zaroxolyn every second or third day
> The patient is a delightful woman in no acute distress.

Needless to say, I particularly enjoy that last comment!

> ASSESSMENT: The patient has class III heart failure symptoms at the present time. Very difficult to balance her fluid status versus her weight. Clearly she did not tolerate going down on her diuretics.

Omana tried to tell him! Ha ha.

After reading half the book Dr. Heywood had recommended, I made a call to Craig in Singapore. I was barely adjusting to the fact that I had congestive heart failure and an ejection fraction of 35%. I started to cry as I paraphrased a sentence from the book: A person can live a reasonably normal life with an EF of 35%.

Craig cut me off gently, saying, "Mom. Mom. You were just fine the last time you called me. It's just a number. Keep enjoying the fun you're having."

I did feel better after talking with my son. I read more of the book, which offered many healthy lifestyle tips. I put the book away without reading the chapter about heart transplants, a subject I assumed had nothing to do with me.

After a few appointments with my new cardiologist I wanted to get something straight in my head. I went over it with him. "I went into the hospital with a strong heart and blocked arteries. I came out with a weakened heart, due to the complications that surfaced during and after surgery. The blocked arteries are now artificially held open with seven stents. Right?" He confirmed that my assessment was correct.

The next three months were filled with commutes from Carlsbad to La Jolla for the Healing Hearts sessions and medical appointments. I chose to travel the Coast Highway, with its beautiful ocean view, instead of the multi-lane freeway most of the time. I had never lived near water before moving to San Diego County. If I had to be sick, at least I was in the best location!

✶ ✶ ✶

The Hidden Messages in Water, a book by Dr. Masaru Emoto, features fascinating photographs of highly magnified water crystals. His amazing photos show crystals with beautiful designs when the water has been exposed to love and certain forms of music. Those same crystals show a chaotic lack of pattern after exposure to cacophonous music or other negative "vibes."

After reading the book and seeing the photographs, I found myself calling out "Hi!" and waving to the ocean as soon as it came into view during my drives. I also drank water from glasses on which I had taped labels bearing the word LOVE. I was following every positive suggestion I was given.

On my way home from appointments, I often stopped to enjoy quiet time in the tranquility of the Self-Realization Fellowship gardens in Encinitas. I went to a meditation session there. As I think you can imagine, I had a hard time sitting in a room filled with interesting people who were silent. I got the itchy-twitchies by the end of the hour. Or maybe it was a half hour. Whichever it was, it was too long for me.

I do benefit from five- to ten-minute quiet times, especially when I add deep breathing. Also, guided meditation has been known to loosen my tight coils for longer periods. When I am tightly coiled, every muscle in my neck and upper back seems to be scrunched up, as if squished into a too-small container. When I close my eyes and concentrate on softening my face and chest with slow, deep breathing, my shoulders start to soften and drop down.

* * *

Yes, 2005 was turning out to be the first time I'd ever felt I was me! I do have good feelings about my roles as mother, wife, sister, grandmother, and teacher. Most self-improvement programs coach you to "be your true self" and then learn to love yourself. I was beginning to do that.

The people-pleasing individuals I have met over the years are quick to say, "I don't know who I am." We are the kind of people who bend toward the people we hope will like us. I just got the image of a plant that leans toward the sun. In some ways, the bending is part of compromising as people work, play, and love together. Compromising is fine if everyone shows respect by honoring each other's interests and values.

This was a year of new friends, activities, and challenges. By June, the highs and lows had become more noticeable. Friends and activities brought the highs. I looked forward to working with my young male trainer; the Healing Hearts members were becoming a close, cohesive group; and girl talk with my friends JoAnn, Sue, and Marilyn A. included stories and fun that had nothing to do with health.

Nevertheless, Dr. Heywood encouraged me to work with a psychologist and see about getting a prescription for an antidepressant. He also told me to take a half dose of the booster diuretic every other day, no matter what weight showed on my scale. I see in my notes that this recommendation came the day after an over-the-top emotional day.

Here's the story on that:

I'd started to cry on the drive to a Healing Hearts session. During the initial taking of our vitals, my tears would not stop. Claire, an RN, offered to walk the track with me so I wouldn't have to go to the exercise room.

Our next activity was the support group session. We knew that Ozzie, our leader, would not be present. However, we were surprised to realize that his substitute was also a no-show. By then, we knew how to run the session. Someone suggested I start our check-in routine, sharing our thoughts about the previous week. I lowered my head and "passed" to the person next to me. I was a quiet listener until it came around to my turn again. I don't remember the words I said as tears rolled down my face. I tried to use polite words to explain a personal problem I had experienced that week.

There was an awkward silence until a fellow came out with words I can't repeat, his version of the cause of my meltdown. Everyone's jaw dropped. He added, "I'm just saying what Linda would say if she wasn't so nice."

I don't remember hearing any other words.

In silence we all headed to a guided meditation and yoga session. I laid my mat down in a back corner. There I sat in a cross-legged pose and let the tears flow. Karen, our teacher, came over, touched me lightly, and then let me have my own quiet time and space.

I did stay for the whole session. Without talking to anyone, I gathered my belongings and walked to my car. I pulled the door closed and sat quietly, trying to gather my composure. Then came the image of my dear Healing Hearts friend saying those outrageous words, followed by that deadly silence. I couldn't help it; I burst out laughing and couldn't stop for the longest time. The next time I saw the tell-it-like-it-is fellow, I gave him a warm hug and thanked him for breaking my dam of fear and anger.

In a group composed of people facing similar struggles, the conversation can get deep and dark. As challenged as my new friends were, they were surprisingly upbeat. We would each tell our personal story and then be shocked by the other stories. While we could share our moments of anger, sadness, or fear, the more cohesive we became, the funnier we got. Hadn't Dr. Heywood told me to laugh more? The Healing Hearts program was proof on so many levels—friendship, love, and laughter—that an integrative approach to medicine can be highly beneficial. It was for me!

✶ ✶ ✶

I know many people have had good experiences with psychologists and psychiatrists. I have always gone in with some kind of bravado and told about my wonderful life, because I was grateful for what I had. The trouble is, I think I gave the impression that I already knew how to handle my concerns. I would be quickly dismissed, without receiving the help, guidance, or push I needed.

Following my doctor's recommendation, I started taking an antidepressant. With no explanation, however, my notes indicate that I stopped taking it just three days later. I must have experienced yucky side effects. I had good non-medical tools for dealing with my emotional roller coaster ride. I'd just have to lean on my strong friend, JoAnn, a bit more often. She didn't fill me with chemicals or hand me a big bill for her services. What a friend! And she lived near me. Best of all, she convinced me that I helped her, too.

When I told my daughter about my bad days, she said, "At least now, Mom, you don't go into a fetal position for three days like you did in the ICU." Every downturn looked better when compared to my setbacks in 2004. Kristin advised me to take a resting day as soon as I realized I was getting too emotional.

At the end of June, I decided to seek out additional groups. I knew the Healing Hearts program would be ending soon. I was invited to attend a nearby church, and one evening I went to an upbeat service. After the service, a nice young woman came over to me. We had a pleasant talk. She said, "It's good that you are looking around." Maybe she had a point.

When I got home, I decided to check the Internet for other worship services in my area. My search was successful, and I felt comfortable in my new niche. I soon joined the women's evening circle, where I met congenial and effervescent women.

As I think about our times together, I find myself smiling. While we had a topic of discussion for each evening, the beginning "check-in sharing" ran the gamut of our latest highs and lows. Laughter snuck in often.

* * *

I made it to my birthday in July. "I'm sixty-five, and I'm alive!" I didn't have a party, but I ran errands wearing a gauzy blouse and a long, swishy skirt. I'd given up on dresses and skirts years ago, but in my girlie attire I felt pretty, happy, grateful, and delighted to have many new friends in San Diego.

> **Hospital Records, June 3, 2005**
>
> Now taking carvedilol, a beta blocker.
>
> No fainting, no defibrillator shocks.
>
> The patient is slowly improving. She is requiring less Zaroxolyn, blood pressure is increasing.
>
> Weight is going up without fluid overload. She will take Zaroxolyn if she goes up two pounds, but only if she feels overtly short of breath.

On July 10th, I went in for a defibrillator (AICD) check. Once again I heard, "You don't use your battery much. That's good." (Do you remember my reaction when I heard a man's story about the first time his AICD did its job? Having learned about the strong jerk a person could feel, I had told the defibrillator in my chest, "Do not go off." So far, so good.)

On July 18th, the medical notes showed that my ejection fraction result was down to 19%. My heart was continuing to lose strength. The accompanying note read, "Extra care with low sodium and fluid intake is not helping."

We started one strong drug that worked directly on the heart muscle to improve its pumping ability, and increased the dose of the beta blocker I was taking to reduce the amount of blood pumped with each heartbeat. They told me my kidneys were being negatively affected, but I don't think I was told the percentage of my ejection fraction.

* * *

During an August appointment with Dr. Heywood, my emotions were better, but I was doing more huffing and puffing. There was some good news: my kidneys were better.

"It's a miracle!" I said.

Dr. Heywood quietly told me, "I prayed for you." Then, in typical Dr. H. style, he said to the fellow (that's a medical title) in the room, "Look at her. She's a babe."

I think it was after that serious and funny visit that I began to refer to Dr. Heywood as "my beloved." To this day, whenever I pop into his secretary's office without an appointment I ask, "Is my beloved here today?" I don't know how he interacted with his other patients. I do know he read me well. He used humor effectively to help me navigate my troubled waters, and I felt safe and well cared for.

It's time to share some of my favorite Dr. Heywood stories. I respect his impeccable credentials. He was giving presentations around the world—unfortunately, often when I needed him most for emotional support. That's when his secretary, Brenda, took over. Brenda had worked with Dr. H. at Loma Linda Hospital, and had accepted his offer to continue working with him in San Diego. She became my go-to person, by phone or in person. She still gives me warm, reassuring hugs!

The more comfortable I grew with Dr. Heywood, the more I became my goofy, talkative self. At the end of one of my appointments I was well into one of my lengthy stories when Dr. H. said, "Linda, I have to go now."

"Okay," I responded, and went back to my story.

"Linda, I really have to go now. Look, I have my hand on the doorknob."

"Go ahead, Dr. Heywood. I'll just talk to the walls."

After that day, they sent a lot of interns, fellows—anybody in a white coat—to the examining room to talk with me before Dr. H. came in. I had the fun of telling funny parts of my story to new ears before the big guy came in to commence with the medical business. I may have been very sick, but I was having the time of my life!

Nurse practitioners can be the strongest link for the patient when it comes to communication. Omana was usually the first person I would see when I arrived. She could decipher my ramblings when I tried to explain what was really happening to me. I'm sure she explained me to the doctors better than I could have explained myself. It was good that she worked with both of my main cardiologists, as she eased my transition from Dr. Rubenson to the new congestive heart failure doctor.

During one of my appointments, after taking my vitals and the initial "So what's going on now?" information, Omana said Dr. H. would be in soon. I told her I had an urgent need to use the bathroom. As I was returning from the bathroom, a loud voice boomed from around the corner. "She's escaped! She's escaped!"

I turned the corner, and there was my tall, crazy doctor. As soon as he spotted me he came over, gave me a big hug, and lifted me in the air. Do you think that caught me off guard? My laughter filled the halls of the clinic.

From then on, Dr. H. had a joke for me at almost every appointment. He is good at telling jokes. Whenever I tried to reciprocate, I would botch up my joke.

"Linda! I think you should have said it this way."

"Oh, right Dr. Heywood, that's the way it really goes."

He could make me laugh, and I could make him groan.

16

I Want Pizza!

Yea! My son's family was home from Singapore, safe and sound. Grace was about to start kindergarten. It was good to know they were close by. It was even better to show them I could handle my medical condition on my own.

In connection with the Healing Hearts program I met Marilyn D., who had done the program a few years earlier. She offered to introduce our group to an interesting stress-reduction technique, commonly called "tapping." The true name is Emotional Freedom Technique (EFT). The goal is to remove negative emotions.

Without trying to explain the technique, I want to share my first experience with it. Since December of 2004, I had wanted to eat pizza. Yes, pizza! With all the fat and salt, the white-flour crust, the deli meat. I had prepared a healthy version that December that turned out to be awful. I was sticking to healthy eating choices, but I lusted for a sinful slice. Why hadn't I allowed myself to eat just a tiny piece? Dumb question. Do you really think I would be satisfied with just one piece?

Back to "tapping": We were asked to think of a negative thought that was causing us stress. The idea was to admit that we had negative thoughts, but to recognize and declare that in spite of them we were still good people. The tapping routine had many steps. On my first attempt I said, "Even though I want to eat unhealthy pizza, I am a good person." I copied Marilyn D.'s tapping pattern while saying the phrase over and over. When we came to a stop, Marilyn asked each one of us how we felt. How strong was our negative emotion or thought now?

I admitted that I still felt bad about wanting the pizza. I added that I was concentrating on doing the tapping correctly more than on taking in the positive thought that I was a good person. During our second round, I was able to focus more on the thought process than on worrying about tapping correctly. In the middle of the routine I got a smile on my face. When the routine was over, Marilyn asked me again how I felt.

Laughing, I explained that the juicy piece of pizza on my mind's TV screen had suddenly disappeared. The smile on my face had come during the tapping, when the pizza image gave way in my mind to an image of the big bags of groceries sitting in the trunk of my car.

On my way to the meeting, I had stopped at a health food store and bought organic spinach, kale, parsley, carrots, Swiss chard, and salt-free tomato juice for my next big batch of the green concoction I drank almost every morning. Where did the pizza go? My negative emotion of guilt had changed to an angelic feeling!

✶ ✶ ✶

The decreasing strength of my heart did not get in the way of good times with my friends. Still, there were a few times when a heavy darkness reduced me to tears when I was alone. In an effort to help me cope with days when I felt useless from fatigue, a psychologist advised me to work with my feeling of uselessness by allowing myself to be comfortable receiving help when I needed it.

In public, I was almost always "up," high on life. If my day was long with appointments or errands, I would start to drag as the day wore on and flop on my bed as soon as possible.

A sweet example was when I stopped one day, late in the afternoon, to pick up a few items at my local grocery store. I don't know how I looked. I became aware that the man behind me was gesturing to the cashier. I don't remember what he said. The gist was that he was concerned about me and wanted the cashier to take note. Together they asked whether I felt okay. Did I need any help? The cashier knew the man behind me, and assured me he could help me out to my car. He offered to follow me home to be sure I arrived there safely.

I told them a bit about my condition. I accepted the help getting my groceries into my car, but declined any further help. I had just a short drive to my home. Once again, I felt I was surrounded by good people. I was tired, but happy to have had that experience.

I told my daughter about the grocery store help and what the psychologist had said about getting a benefit from the "useless" feeling. Her comment started with, "Mom, how do you feel when you help someone?" I said I felt good, happy to help. "Then give that gift to someone else. Let others help you." Her comment rang in my ears. It made it much easier to admit I could use some help—but just on my bad days.

Around this time I began a close relationship with Diane, a woman in the evening women's group I had joined. At an event we both attended she made the comment, "I think we have made a connection." Indeed, we had. We began to meet for dinner before the evening meetings. We soon realized we had a lot in common. Little did I know then how big a role she was to play in my life the next year.

* * *

In the fall I started another diuretic. Would we ever find a medicine that would prevent the fluid buildup and not cause horrid side effects?

In my struggle to get a good night's sleep, I tried taking a sleeping aid. In the middle of one night, I woke up feeling hungry. I decided to go to my kitchen and have a rice cracker with peanut butter. When I got to the kitchen I found the crackers, the peanut butter, and a sticky knife on the table. It seems I had been there earlier.

Another night, I heard a funny sound. The next morning, I found a broken ceramic vase on the floor on the far side of my bed. I must have walked over there and bumped the shelf.

The peanut butter incident convinced me to stop taking that sleeping aid. Even if I had to start taking a nap in the afternoon, that would be preferable to taking another drug. The funny thing was that my friend Marilyn A., who was dealing with MS, had been prescribed drugs similar to ones I'd tried for anxiety, depression, and sleep. We talked about becoming "druggies." We laughed about it, but we did not like that image. Sharing our fears made us stronger, more able to handle our bad days with as few drugs as possible.

One wonderful way to get a good night's sleep was to set an appointment with Kari, a massage therapist. She would bring her massage table in the late afternoon or early evening. I remember the easing of tension as she massaged me. I also think fondly of the conversations we enjoyed.

* * *

I did my first American Heart Association San Diego Heart Walk in September, 2005. The national organization uses their donations to help improve patient care, fund lifesaving research, and educate people at risk of developing cardiovascular disease.

I went by myself. It was not long before I saw several Healing Hearts staff members. I walked the "Survivor's Route" with Derek and his friend until they took off on the longer walk. I felt so good when I finished the shorter walk that I decided to walk the longer route. But when the road led uphill, I had no trouble changing my mind and doubling back.

* * *

The next day, I was off on another trip. This time I was flying to Spokane. Kristin drove from their new home in Idaho to pick me up. The long drive gave us a chance to talk about this new chapter in her life. Brian was starting his teaching career as a research professor at a university in Idaho.

It was good to see their new home, and we had interesting adventures in the beautiful rural area. I felt healthy out in the crisp air. We walked up a hill to a park that was perfect for the family dogs.

My favorite memory is of cuddling with my grandson when he became uneasy waiting for his parents to return from a date night. There is nothing better than having your grandson snuggle and feel safe in your arms.

Distraction was good for me. I learned that being with my family and friends turned off the uneasy thoughts that came when I was home alone.

Before the year ended I took a third trip, this time with college friends. Judy, Ann, and I had celebrated our sixtieth birthdays together and had agreed to celebrate our sixty-fifth together as well. We had hoped to visit Taos, New Mexico, but upon checking with my doctor I learned that the high altitude would not be good for me.

Instead, Tucson, Arizona, became our destination. It really didn't matter where we went. We talked like magpies and laughed like hyenas whenever we were together. We enjoyed a nice motel, good food, and interesting excursions. My heart problem did not get in the way of having fun. We just chose our activities carefully. I did accept the suggestion to use a wheelchair at a desert preserve.

Grace's birthday was celebrated in the fall. Many friends and family members arrived to honor the five-year-old. She looked so grown up to me.

Parties at my son's home were such a contrast to the parties we'd had when my kids were growing up. I had been a nervous hostess. Both of my kids entertain easily. With the help of their spouses, they set a casual, playful, and well-prepared atmosphere.

Thanksgiving, Christmas, and New Year's Eve were good but uneventful celebrations.

Would 2006 be the year with no obstacles? The future is always uncertain, isn't it. Just in case, fasten your roller coaster seat belt!

17

Consistently Inconsistent in 2006

I had kept my promise to myself to live a healthy lifestyle. I'd eaten carefully, watched my fluids and sodium intake, exercised with a trainer, walked a lot, and learned the value of support groups and deep friendships. My heart was not strong, yet I had stayed active.

After the bustle of the holidays, I experienced a slight dip in my energy level. A major happy distraction came with a visit from my daughter and grandson. Of the many activities we enjoyed, my favorite was watching Aengus, two and a half years old, interact with Grace, five, and Tori, almost four. They devised their own activities. So precious!

Now that I was back to being alone, I found it easier to control food preparation. Super-low-sodium, low-fat, low-sugar meals could be achieved by eating individual pieces of fruit, vegetables, and bits of chicken, rather than adding the extra ingredients found in recipes. I used spray margarine and spray salad dressings to cut calories. My goal was to eat the lowest-calorie foods with dense nutritional value, the "super foods"— blueberries, kiwi, spinach, kale, avocados, nuts, yogurt, and so on.

I spent hours washing, cutting, and simmering green vegetables and carrots to make my healthy green morning drink. I pureed the greens. I often did the prep in the evening, ending up exhausted and leaving myself with dirty pots, blender, and olive-green splotches on the stove and counter.

Years later, I would buy a high-power super blender. Why didn't someone introduce me to that time-saving machine while I had congestive heart failure?

Before I could force myself to drink my green juice, I had to heat it with salt-free tomato juice to make it palatable. I couldn't get JoAnn to take a sip. "I can't get past the awful color," she groaned.

My trainer, Joel, and I worked well together. I didn't feel much stronger, but I had improved at stretching, doing balance work, and using weights.

My young trainers always wanted to call me "ma'am." Yuck. I knew they were showing respect. Still … Yuck! I told Joel, "Watch out. I will slug you if you say 'ma'am' again."

At some point Joel moved to a gym farther from my home. I went there for my private sessions with him and did extra aerobic work at my local gym. In two different gyms I became known as "Slugger," Joel's name for me. I may have blushed, but I loved walking by the good-looking guys and hearing them call out, "Hey, Slugger. How's it going?"

✳ ✳ ✳

Remember Marilyn D., the woman who introduced me to "tapping"? She had helped me see that I was a vital part of my medical team. I had to do my part so the doctors could more effectively do their work.

She and Claire had taken special training that soon impacted the lives of many women in the greater San Diego area. By mid-year, they had introduced me to WomenHeart, The National Coalition for Women with Heart Disease.

WomenHeart's mission is to improve the health and quality of life of women living with or at risk of heart disease, and to advocate for our benefit. By 2015, the organization had trained close to seven hundred female heart disease survivors as community educators via the WomenHeart Science & Leadership Symposium, in collaboration with Mayo Clinic.

Claire led a WomenHeart group in La Jolla. Later, Marilyn D. started her group in Carlsbad. I missed the first meeting, but have been a member ever since. I am quick to admit that I attended my first meeting just to support Marilyn. Although the idea of entering a room filled with women who were fearful about heart disease hadn't sounded appealing, I was surprised to find that I felt comfortable from the beginning.

As time went on, regularly attending members began to feel a sisterly bond. We truly cared about each other. Via email, Marilyn would alert us to a member's upcoming surgery or a personal concern that could benefit from kind and optimistic words from other members.

I loved the sense of humor that developed in the group. Some sessions got pretty heavy, yet even little bits of humor could help us see the bigger picture of the ups and downs that come on the roller coaster ride of life.

From the national headquarters came the distribution of Red Bags of Courage, with pertinent heart disease information for women. Marilyn and Suzie, another WomenHeart educator, had come up with the idea of including a red HeartScarf knitted by loving volunteers.

The idea was well received and implemented. A woman in our area had recently celebrated completion of one thousand red scarves, only to begin work on her next thousand. That's a lot of knitting! Her husband had experienced two heart attacks and surgery. She knew what our members were going through.

I wore my scarf to WomenHeart gatherings as well as to medical procedures. We wanted medical personnel to be aware of the support patients could receive if they knew about our organization. Wouldn't it be awesome if doctors would give their women patients a WomenHeart pamphlet right after they informed them about their heart issue?!

* * *

My neighbors formed a group I chose to call "Condo Crazies." It took the arrival of our new neighbor, Sherin, to draw us closer in friendship. Not long after he moved in, he suggested that we go out to brunch once in a while. A few of us took the bait. Soon the group included all the neighbors in our short cul-de-sac and their guests.

* * *

In April, I learned about the birth of Petra, my newest granddaughter. I was with my great-niece, Ariana, when my daughter called to let me know she was in labor but not yet ready to go to the hospital We were celebrating Ari's birthday a day late. Kristin's labor was extremely short this time, unlike her very long labor with Aengus.

I learned that Kristin and Brian arrived at the hospital just in time to get to a delivery room. My daughter called me again, barely four hours later, to announce Petra's birth. "What just happened?" was Brian's reaction to the speed and ease of this birth. (During Kristin's pregnancy, I told her I had experienced another vision with the message that she would have an easier labor this time. My vision, once again, had been accurate!)

* * *

On April 25th, I had an interview to see whether I would qualify for a clinical study involving defibrillators. I was asked several questions and told details regarding the study. When Dr. Heywood came in, I mentioned that I felt the same tingling in my left arm I had occasionally experienced from the late '90s up to the time of my bypass surgery. Whoa. Stop the presses. I could not proceed with the study. "Nothing can be going on at the start of the study," he said, "but you might be considered at a later date."

Since I could not be in the study, I wouldn't have a nuclear cardiology stress test. I had hoped to have the test before my trip to Idaho to see my new granddaughter. The problem of my weight, my need for diuretics, and the pressure in my ribs remained.

Dr. Heywood said he would order a different test I could have before my trip. But on the day of that test, the nurse saw that I had already had a similar test too recently. No test.

Now, Dr. H. was in hot water. I stormed over to his office. "I know," he said. "I'm in big trouble for not remembering that other test."

"You need to do some major damage repair work on me," I retorted. Swish! Once again he'd picked me up. This time, he added twirling. How could I stay mad when I was laughing so hard?

An angiogram was scheduled to be done right after my trip to Idaho. Dr. H. said, "We do need to see what is going on in there."

* * *

I had a wonderful visit with Kristin's family the first week in May. The opportunity to spend time with my newest granddaughter brought tender, calming memories of the first time I'd held each of my children and grandchildren.

* * *

The angiogram on May 12th showed two clogged stents. Two new stents were inserted. I also started on a new medicine regime, including an antiplatelet to inhibit blood clots and a new cholesterol-lowering drug. I drove to Craig's home and spent the night there.

In the morning, I was surprised to hear that my Mothers Day gift was to be a trip to visit beautiful local flower fields with Craig and the girls. It was a gorgeous day, but hot. We did a lot of walking, quite a feat for someone who'd had an angiogram the day before.

* * *

To be in tip-top condition for my second trip to Idaho, I got two injections to help my ailing back. As my doctor was looking at my weak left foot and ankle, she noticed a bad rash. "Most likely caused by an arthritis flare-up," she said. "Those shots I gave you should help get rid of it." A medical two-fer. Yep. The rash was soon gone! Now, what to do for the cold I'd picked up the day before?

The next day, Omana prescribed an inhaler to help with my increasing breathlessness. My cold was not going away. Since she was aware that I was heading back to Idaho the next day for my grandson's third birthday celebration, she wanted me to take an antibiotic.

The last week in May I was again flying north. My back pain was gone by the time I arrived, and my leg felt better. The shots were doing their job. Distraction was a big factor, I'm sure.

Our restaurant breakfast with fancy pancakes was a big hit with the birthday boy, followed by a party with one of Kristin's specialty cakes. This time the kids enjoyed eating a fancy tractor on delicious dirt. I loved watching the little guests politely line up to receive their piece of cake. The roomful of people talking and laughing gave me yet another sweet image to store away in my memory and pull out when I was alone at home.

I soon realized I felt the best I had since the beginning of the year—no back, foot, ankle, or knee pain, no wheezing, and no breathlessness. I had more energy than I had felt recently.

The energy held up when I returned home on June 5th, and my weight remained in a surprisingly good range. I felt well enough to do a physical therapy session and work out with Joel. Have I mentioned that I always choose to work with good-looking young men? If I have to exercise, I should get some personal benefit!

At my June 9th appointment, Omana said the better energy and breathing were signs that the stents were working. My AICD check showed no blips and no battery usage, meaning I had not needed the use of the pacemaker or defibrillator. That was all good news.

✶ ✶ ✶

Kristin brought Aengus and Petra for a visit in July. I took advantage of the opportunity for a "photo op" with all four of my grandchildren. Craig's family was about to leave for another year in Singapore. Filled with fond memories of their last experience, they had signed up to go again to represent the company.

✶ ✶ ✶

In early August of 2006, I learned that I did not qualify for another clinical study because my heart was too healthy. My latest echo showed an ejection fraction of 40%. Good news! Much better than when I left the hospital.

As far as I can remember and according to what I've seen in my personal notes, I was not told the results of the several echocardiograms that were done after I left the hospital. The medical records I requested years later showed an EF of 20% in May of 2005. The jump to 40% was more impressive than I had imagined.

* * *

Uh oh. The next day, I started to feel dizzy. I got low numbers when I took my blood pressure. The tightness in my chest worsened as the day wore on. I called my insurance company's night nurse line, and the nurse who answered insisted I call an ambulance. I really didn't want to; I guess I was embarrassed. When I talked to the dispatcher, I pleaded with her to tell them not to use the siren.

I was able to go to my front door, so they didn't have to bash it in. I had worked myself into quite a state. "Lady, calm down," they said. "You did the right thing." (I remember hearing that several times.)

After examining me in the ER, they decided to keep me overnight. There was no new heart event. I think my nerves had gotten out of hand. That's when I was told to take a relaxing drug to help with anxiety tension.

Later that month, I had a urinary infection that was easily treated. We stopped one of my drugs because I was gaining weight too fast while trying to wait longer between booster diuretic days. Dr. Heywood began saying frequently, "Linda, you are consistently inconsistent!"

Most days, I was able to do a forty-minute walk. One warm evening, JoAnn and I had a good talk as we walked together. On the way back I stopped, realizing I would not be able to walk the rest of the way home. It was getting dark, and JoAnn made sure I had a safe place to sit before she went back to get her car. (A long time later, she would admit to having practically run home, filled with fear. I don't remember being afraid. For once, I was being realistic about my limitations.)

In an email to my friend Ron, I told him about another walk. I had put off taking my doozie diuretic. "I did my full walk, but with tons of stops along the way," I wrote. "My left arm was quite tingly. The tingling went away as soon as I got home, and I began to feel better all over." I got a quick response from my caring protector, telling me to be sure to retell my story to my physicians, including all the details.

On Friday, September 6th, I had a day with terrible pressure in my rib cage. I couldn't sleep that night. I finally gave up and took a booster diuretic. Not long before, I had been able to wait five to six days before taking the doozie diuretic. This time only three days had passed. It happened again that I had to take a dose after just three days, and on the 11th I had to take one after only two days.

At my congestive heart failure appointment with Omana on September 15th, my blood pressure readings were good. My oxygen rate was 94%, but I had found it difficult to walk from the parking garage to the clinic. I could manage only shallow breathing.

✷ ✷ ✷

I had my first non-medical outing with Dr. Heywood over the weekend. I had already planned to do my second American Heart Association San Diego Heart Walk on September 16th. Dr. H decided he wanted to walk with his patients. He ordered special T-shirts for us.

I arrived at the crack of dawn. I had taken my doozie diuretic, and hoped to use the "sweet-smelling Port-a-Potties" a few times before the Walk. I was feeling a lot of pressure in my ribs, but I knew that happy distractions worked wonders for me. The commotion of the loud, lively crowd lifted my spirits.

The Walk began with the Red Hat "heart disease survivors," who had experienced heart complications or serious procedures and had been given red caps to wear during the walk. We walked, talked, and laughed as we traversed the short route. All around us were the more capable walkers and runners who were going the longer distance. At age sixty-five, I was not the oldest member of our group. To my surprise, however, I was the one who slowed down our pace. I'd had a much easier time the previous year.

At one point, I stopped. Dr. Heywood turned and asked, "Are you all right?" I paused, and then did a big swallowing action that had nothing to do with sipping water. I guess I took a big breath at the same time, though I hadn't felt short of breath. After one "swallow," I resumed walking.

Once again, I stopped and repeated the previous action. Dr. H. looked somewhat alarmed. "Do you need to sit down?" he asked.

"No. I'm fine." I did the swallow action again. "Okay. Let's go."

I remember stopping only twice. This stopping and swallowing action was typical for me on long walks on high-fluid days. I was not alarmed about having to stop a couple of times. I had learned to listen to my body and do what was necessary to reduce stress.

Walking with my doctor and some of his other patients was a unique and enjoyable experience. Dr. Heywood entertained us with his corny jokes, and the laughter made it fun. Many patients might as well have been in camouflage gear, so well did they blend in with non-patients in this non-hospital setting.

18

A Whole New Adventure Begins

On September 18th, two days after the San Diego Heart Walk, I went to work out with Joel. I had taken a booster diuretic, but felt no relief. Joel suggested we just take a walk. We quickly discovered that walking was more painful than working with weights indoors.

At the gym I received a call from Dr. Heywood. He said he wanted me to go to the hospital the next day. He told me I should have someone take me.

My mind started to take off in several directions. My roller coaster ride was becoming erratic. At times I seemed to be improving. Memories of times with my grandchildren danced in my head as I did my daily walking.

Then the constant pressure I felt in my stomach and chest would tug at my pleasant thoughts, casting a dark cloud over them. The zig-zagging mental exercises took me to conflicting images of my long stay in the ICU back in 2004. I smiled when I envisioned the sweet interchanges I'd enjoyed with my medical team, but then the reality of the scary twists and turns would take center stage.

I don't think I was worried about what they would find. I just hoped they would find out what was causing the pressure. It might not be my heart. I was more worried about all the possible errors and complications that could arise. During phone calls to Kristin and Craig, I promised I would go to sleep with outrageously positive thoughts.

I arrived at Scripps Green Hospital on the 19th for a visit that would last until the 26th. My notes about that week are sketchy.

In an attempt to deal with my nervousness about going back to the hospital, I prepared an eight-and-a-half-by-eleven-inch paper to show anyone who would be working with me:

Handle With Care

Linda S. LeVier 7-7-1940 66 years old

first experience with heart problems

was in March 2004

I do feel that I am in good hands. I truly love my doctors and the staff in the ICU. They brought me through a very difficult medical situation. They witnessed the many complications I experienced.

I want all of you to be very careful to follow all the proper procedures. If you wonder at my fear, just look at my right leg. Bandages were left on too long after my bypass and stent operations. I think I almost lost my leg.

Yes, I admit, hospitals scare me. I have plans to live a very long life. I have two children and four precious grandchildren I have to watch over for many years. By the way, you are all invited to my 107th birthday party!

Hospital Records, September 20, 2006

Entered with info from a cardiac stress test that showed negative for ischemia, and an EF of 21%. Chief complaint: dyspnea on exertion (shortness of breath) and abdominal/epigastric pressure/ tightness even after eating a few bites.

Esophagogastroduodenoscopy: (Upper Endoscopy/EGD) to examine lining of esophagus for digestive problems, structural or functional abnormalities.

Reason for GI Consultation: Early satiety and abdominal discomfort; ultrasound showed no ascites, right pleural effusion, normal liver, no gallbladder wall thickening, no gall stones.

There were no new findings. There was no gastric pathology, no known cause for my abdominal discomfort. I was told to continue taking my regular diuretic and the booster diuretic every day.

Three days after I left the hospital, I was back in Scripps Green Hospital—from September 29th to October 2nd, 2006.

I don't have personal notes from that hospital visit. My bad days were becoming more frequent, with weight gain, discomfort, and labored breathing.

✳ ✳ ✳

I can't emphasize enough the warmth and encouragement I felt from the women in WomenHeart and my evening circle. They bolstered my spirits and courage during the rough patches of my journey.

Yes, women talk a lot, but they can also be compassionate listeners. They let you cry. They give warm hugs. I know now that I stay emotionally healthier when caring and strong women are in my life.

I'd like to share bits of an email I received from one of my Healing Hearts women supporters:

"I'm sending lots of positive energy, smiles, and good old-fashioned stubbornness your way …. I've always enjoyed your perky, feisty, positive presence in our circle, and your love of laughter always makes me smile."

With that kind of support, what could possibly go wrong?

✳ ✳ ✳

On October 5th, I learned that Craig was coming from Singapore to take care of some work locally. I was happy to know I would soon see him.

On October 6th, driving down the coast on my way to my Congestive Heart Failure Clinic appointment, I decided to ask Omana whether I might qualify for a handicapped parking placard. I would use it only on my bad days.

During the initial exam, Omana said she would get the parking placard paperwork ready for me. In came Dr. Heywood. He sat down, which was uncharacteristic of him. After giving his approval for my handicapped placard, he said, "Linda, my team and I have been reviewing your condition and all of the medications and tests we have done. We believe you would benefit from having a heart transplant."

I remember saying, in surprise, "Dr. Heywood, you must think I am very sick! That hadn't occurred to me."

No, I did not sob, though I did let a few tears escape down my cheeks. Dr. H. said, "I knew you'd cry. I told my wife this morning, 'She will cry, but I have to tell her because I really care for her.'"

I hope Dr. H. remembers that I came around quickly after we discussed the reason I needed a heart transplant. I asked how long I might live without one. I believe I heard that I might live two to three years, but that I would have more bad days and they would be closer together. I quickly gave my consent.

By the time I was driving home, I was excited about letting go of part of the medical history on my father's side of my family. My father, his father, his brother and sister, and one of my sisters had all had heart problems. Our conditions varied at the start, but our hearts were what gave way at the end.

During my drive home, my mind fixated on the great new plan for my condition. I don't remember being afraid of the radical surgery. I switched my thinking to the email from Craig. What amazing timing! Craig would probably be able to meet Dr. Heywood. Together we could ask all the important questions. I began to think about the phone calls I would soon make to Kristin and Craig.

There was no way I could be alone with this huge, unexpected information. Thank goodness, JoAnn was at home. As soon as I sat down, the tears spilled, a mixture of happy and oh-my-gosh tears. JoAnn was the best person for me to talk to that Friday.

It was a few minutes before 5:00pm when my cell phone rang. There I was, sitting on JoAnn's couch. The voice on the phone said, "I'm Vicki, from Dr. Jaski's office." I barely remembered that Dr. Heywood had told me about Dr. Jaski, who would be an excellent heart transplant cardiologist for me. Dr. H. had said that Dr. Jaski would be my new favorite doctor. "No one can replace you," I had whined.

(Why couldn't Dr. H. be my heart transplant cardiologist? Because heart transplants were not performed at Scripps Green Hospital. Instead, the surgery would be done by a Sharp Memorial Hospital surgeon and Dr. Jaski would be my pre- and post-transplant cardiologist. I would continue to see Dr. Heywood, my primary congestive heart failure cardiologist.)

Vicki had a nice manner. The sound of her voice calmed me. She must have asked about several things, but I only remember hearing something about health insurance. After a few minutes, she called again to inform me that although insurance or lack thereof could bring undue stress to a medical situation, I needn't worry, as my insurance would cover my transplant procedure and medicines.

JoAnn and I couldn't believe I had received two calls from Dr. Jaski's office so soon after learning that I needed a heart transplant. Vicki's words and tone had been unbelievably reassuring to this excited and very nervous transplant candidate. I'd known instantly that I was going to have a caring new medical team.

The calls to Kristin and Craig went well. They both remembered hearing in 2004 that a heart transplant might be a possibility down the line. I don't think I'd been given that information. My son was particularly good about sensing what facts I could handle. While they both promised to support my wishes, my kids made it clear that the final decision to give the "okay" for a heart transplant had to be mine.

During my call to Craig, I told him that Dr. Heywood wanted to meet with him. The appointment was set for the 13th.

As my son and I approached the clinic, Craig said he might like to talk to Dr. Heywood alone. I countered by saying that this time I was ready and interested to know all the facts and concerns.

Dr. Heywood discussed my changing medical condition. He told us about the different medicines, tests, and procedures they had tried. A heart transplant would not be considered until all other options had been exhausted. Then he began to tell Craig about what had happened during the San Diego Heart Walk. Wide-eyed, he stated, "She scared me!"

We discussed heart transplantation from all angles, the benefits and the possible complications, for forty-five minutes. Craig and I were ready to learn about my next steps. While confident I was making the correct decision, I felt reassured when Craig was satisfied with Dr. Heywood's answers and explanations. It was a definite "Yes" from me.

In an email to my friends Ron and Vicki, I shared some of the comments from the meeting with Dr. Heywood. He had told me to keep doing the things that felt good. He definitely wanted me to keep walking, and he gave me the go-ahead to continue working with my trainer, Joel.

In my email, I added, "My spirits are good, but of course there is a little fear lurking around. I can't believe the huge local support I am gathering."

Two nights earlier, I had talked to a young mother I'd met in the WomenHeart group. Her heart problem had begun during her pregnancy, and her EF score had dropped to 10% after the birth of her son. Nine days after she was accepted into the program, Cathleen had received a new heart. That had been in January of that same year, 2006. She looked and sounded so good.

The appointment to meet Dr. Jaski was set for October 19th. I told my WomenHeart friends I was about to be screened for acceptance as a heart transplant patient. After the meeting, Marilyn D. offered to go with me to meet the doctor. Another member, Kathy, also offered to go along. I hadn't had time to think about going alone, though my son had returned to Singapore.

Sitting quietly that evening at home, I realized what an immense sense of relief I felt knowing that I would be surrounded by love and calmness in my first meeting with my transplant cardiologist. I was approaching a serious twist in my health journey. It is always good to have extra ears to retain the medical information given to patients, especially when the doctor and procedure are in a totally unfamiliar realm.

October 19th was a life-changing day for me. While Marilyn drove, Kathy worked her de-stressing magic on me. She and Marilyn were determined to unwind my tightly coiled neck and shoulders.

I knew I was in good hands after seeing and talking with Dr. Jaski and Vicki, his nurse practitioner. The doctor gave me lots of information and answered all our questions. He told us about one of their women patients who had just celebrated twenty years with her transplanted heart.

In my nervousness, I said I had read somewhere that age sixty-five was the outer limit for accepting a heart transplant candidate. I quickly added that I was a very young sixty-six. I'm quite sure he said, "Yes, I've heard about you." The rest of the visit remains a blur, except that I do recall receiving some printed information about heart transplantation.

I had lab tests that day. I counted sixteen vials filled with my blood! The nurse switched smoothly from one vial to the next. It was the least painful draw I'd ever had.

Kathy, Marilyn, and I returned to the car and let out our excitement. Marilyn and Kathy were as impressed as I was with my new medical team. I was growing excited about what was to come.

✱ ✱ ✱

Kathy offered to come to my home and help me learn how to work with HeartMath techniques. She taught me how to do some exercises that utilized rhythmic breathing while consciously shifting my negative thoughts to positive thoughts. I was learning how to neutralize the effects of stress on my body. As I began to fully realize the seriousness of my heart condition, I was grateful to have a variety of stress-reducing tools. Keeping my heart safe became a top priority in deciding how to use my time.

Continuing to get out and mix with upbeat people kept my spirits high most of the time. Practicing the rhythmic breathing and the tapping system Marilyn D. had taught me, plus believing that I could choose my attitude, helped me feel I was being proactive in managing my health.

The researchers at HeartMath write about a personal coherence that refers to the synchronization of our physical, mental, and emotional systems. This coherence can be measured by our heart rhythm patterns: The more balanced and smooth they are, the more in sync, or coherent, we are. Stress levels recede, energy levels increase, and our brain and what Heart-Math calls the "heart brain" work together.

✱ ✱ ✱

My next hurdle would be to pass the medical tests that would determine whether I would be an acceptable heart transplant candidate. I was to be at the hospital for pre-transplant testing by 7:00 on the morning of October 24th. Was there some way to cram for those tests? How sick did I have to be?

I believed I had to be sick enough in some areas and well enough in others. Talk about pressure! I was to stay two nights in the hospital. They said they would let me know before I went home whether I had been accepted to receive a heart transplant.

I had planned to drive my car to the test. I hated to put anyone out, especially at that time of the morning. A couple of friends had offered to drive me. Kathy, who had gone with me to meet Dr. Jaski, had told me I could change my mind and call for a ride up to one hour before I would need her to pick me up.

I agonized over my decision. Finally, I decided I shouldn't drive myself home after all the tests. If I did get accepted I would be overjoyed, but nervous. I would not be fit for driving. If I did not get accepted, I would be distraught, thinking I had but two to three years to live without the hope of receiving a new heart. I would definitely not be fit for driving!

I gave in and called Kathy the night before the test. She insisted she was an early-morning person. I felt so relieved that I may even have slept a little that night. I got up, took a shower, and pulled out clean clothes. What? Didn't your mother tell you to be sure to always wear clean underwear? "You never know what will happen in your day," mine always said. So there I was, looking for clothes in the dim light of early morning. Why hadn't I laid everything out the night before? I don't know.

Kathy arrived right on time. Leaving so early in the morning meant we were graced with decent traffic. At the hospital I thanked her for her kindness, sent her on her way, and walked into the lobby to get checked in. Soon I was taken to my room. It was time to put on a hospital gown.

As I reached down to take off my socks I gasped, "Oh no! I'm wearing purple socks. I didn't even know I had purple socks." I thought of my mother and how embarrassed she would have been. She would have wanted to call a cab to go home and change. (Remember, I had dismissed my driver.)

I am not my mother. Instead of freaking out, I laughed, and the nurse laughed along with me. In fact, all of the medical personnel I saw that day laughed with me. The purple socks I'd forgotten I owned turned out to be the icebreaker before each test.

One of the tests, of course, involved a treadmill. I was already in my bright purple socks and a floppy hospital gown that opened in the back. Someone handed me green hospital pants to wear. One of the fellows said, "Yes, one size that fits no one."

Just before the test was to begin, I was given a clear plastic tube to put in my mouth. It was fat and bent, and placing it properly was difficult. It would measure the amount of oxygen I used as I walked.

I looked absolutely charming. Before I could think to be embarrassed, I heard another fellow say, "Where's a camera when we need one?" Right.

I busted up with laughter. I then had to try once more to get that big tube into my mouth and stop thinking funny thoughts. This was serious. I had to qualify to get on the heart transplant list!

I was at Sharp Memorial Hospital for a few days more than I had anticipated. There were more tests and a talk with a social worker and a psychologist, as I recall.

Yes! I got the important answer. I would soon be on the official waiting-for-a-heart-transplant list! They told me I would get my pager when I stopped taking one of my medicines.

I told you the lengthy story about those crazy purple socks because they had taken on a life of their own. I was told to be sure to wear them when I went to the hospital for my surgery. Someone said purple was a spiritual color, and the socks would be sure to help bring about a successful surgical outcome. I had several opportunities to wear the socks before and after the surgery. They became a staple at medical appointments and support groups.

Later, I found I had not one but two pairs of purple socks. I finally remembered that they'd been given to me on my airline flights to and from Singapore. The flights were long, and those comfortable socks beat wearing shoes the whole time. One pair of socks went into my hospital bag, waiting for "The Call." The other pair stayed in my sock drawer.

Jim, my financial adviser and the dear friend who had helped me connect with the Healing Hearts program, drove me home that day. During the drive to my home he commented, "I can't wait for an invitation to your 'I'm Okay' party."

A few days later, Sherin, the condo group instigator, stopped by for a short visit. He brought me flowers. My heart problem had brought a big boost to my social life.

My spirits had risen as my fear about my condition had lessened. I told my daughter I thought having the safety net of doctors from two hospitals watching me had made me stronger emotionally.

Both my daughter and son knew I had been accepted for transplantation. It was time to tell my two nephews, Chris and Jeff, whose mother (my sister Jean) had died at the young age of forty. In October of 1968, she had been offered a heart transplant option as a last resort to save her life.

Dr. Christiaan Barnard from South Africa had worked with Dr. Shumway at Stanford University Hospital. Heart transplantation was in its infancy. The first heart transplant in the United States had been performed by Dr. Shumway on January 6th, 1968. While the operations were going well, keeping patients alive after the operation was a mystery. Patients were living barely days to weeks in 1968.

Jean had not given her consent for the experimental surgery. Jeff told me his mother would have been Stanford Hospital's thirty-seventh heart transplant recipient. She died in October of 1968. My sister had suffered from an undiagnosed illness for most of her life. The medical community never figured out how to help her.

I held a sad memory of Jean's short life, for she hadn't had the joy of watching her sixteen- and ten-year-old sons become good men. Chris and Jeff are both fathers. I choose to believe that Jean is in a beautiful place, watching her sons, grandchildren, and great-grandchildren charm the rest of us. I'm sure she is proud of them and all they have accomplished.

My father and I had heart problems unrelated to what Jean endured. While I never forgot about her heart transplant possibility, I did not grow older under a dark cloud. Now I had the difficult task of telling my nephews I would soon be on the waiting list to receive a new heart. Yet when I told them the news, they each made optimistic comments without hesitation. "You will be fine, Aunt Linda ... there has been so much progress in the field of heart transplants ... keep up your good attitude!"

November 2nd turned out to be an interesting day. I chose that day to call my sister Marilyn with my latest information. Jeff and his daughter arranged to be at my sister's home when I called. Marilyn took the news well. I kept telling her how excited I was about the possibility of receiving a new heart. After the call, Jeff and Ari took her out to dinner to give her a chance to share her thoughts with them.

As for me, I was about to attend my first meeting with heart transplant recipients.

19

Expanding Community Support

I was invited by my WomenHeart friend Cathleen to go to the Sharp Memorial Hospital Heart Transplant Support Group. For good luck, I wore my purple socks and my WomenHeart red HeartScarf that evening.

While walking from the parking lot, Cathleen (the young mother who had received her new heart that year) kept looking back at me as I hurried to catch up to her. In a short time, she had progressed from not being able to carry her baby from one room to another to easy walking. I found that inspiring.

I was surprised to see a big group of people. We watched a video, "The Sharp Experience," highlighting a heart transplant story. There in front of me, on a big screen, I watched the heart transplant surgery and heard the facts. When the video was over, someone asked me how I felt after seeing "everything" during my first meeting. Before I could answer, the man next to me called out, "She was fascinated. She leaned forward and watched every detail!"

I soon realized I had gained yet another group of understanding new friends. As the meeting was drawing to a close, a group member told me that most meetings were not as rowdy as was this one. Please, the rowdiness wasn't my fault. I was the nervous first-timer. True, my loud laughing may have encouraged some of the people to laugh loudly. At home that night, I relived the fun I'd had with these people brought together by a serious life challenge.

✳ ✳ ✳

I continued taking walks, working out with Joel, and handling my domestic chores. I was tiring more quickly now and was obliged to stop and rest more often.

On that note, let me tell you about a special event I attended on November 5th. Before learning that I needed a new heart, I had received an invitation to the wedding of my friend Barbara's son. Our friendship dated back to Lamaze childbirth-preparation classes. The young groom had been born four days after my daughter, Kristin, and our families had stayed in touch over the years. Barbara's daughter had married a few years earlier, but I had been unable to attend her wedding. I was determined not to miss this one. I had sent my RSVP, saying I was looking forward to attending the special event.

Once I learned that I would soon be on the waiting-for-a-heart list, I called Barbara. The wedding would be just before I was to be added to the list. I felt comfortable with the idea of driving from Carlsbad to San Juan Capistrano, a little over an hour's drive. I laughed when I told her that I might already have my pager by that time, but that I would not get a call that night.

The late-afternoon wedding was in a lovely location. I was pleased I hadn't let my declining health keep me from sharing this beautiful occasion with my friend.

After the wedding, I found my table and sat down for dinner. A man asked, "Do you have your pager?" I made a funny face and asked whether he knew why I would have a pager. As it turned out, I had been placed at a table with Barbara's relatives, who had been informed of my condition and given the responsibility of watching over me.

The evening was filled with good food, music, and conversation. I took just one tiny sip of champagne during a wedding toast. One promise I had made to the transplant team was to stay away from alcohol and cigarettes. I had never been a smoker, but I did drink wine once in a while. Still, it would be no problem skipping wine while I waited for a new heart. My cardiologist had given me permission to have the tiny taste of champagne.

As the evening wore on, the music and dancing revved up—and so did I. After 8:00, I couldn't sit still. I got up and started dancing with several young girls. A couple of men danced with me. I was one of the last ones to leave the party, still totally keyed up.

Driving home down the coast freeway under the dark, starry sky, with a big smile on my face, I reached a point where all I could see were ocean ripples, low hillsides, and the other cars on the freeway. Out of the blue, I slowly began to unravel. I don't think I had trouble breathing until after I pictured myself dancing so joyfully. Then the fear struck me that I was alone, with a life-threatening condition, driving at freeway speed.

I tried to calm myself with deep breathing and thinking happy thoughts about the wedding. Then crept in the horror of what would happen to Barbara if I died on the way home from her son's wedding. I moved to the slow lane and drove extra-carefully. I thought the drive took forever, but I got home in record time.

Fully aware of how anxiety builds in me, I took an anti-anxiety pill when I arrived home. I sat on the edge of my bed and called my insurance company's nurse line. I began to calm down as I filled a nurse in on the full story. Since I was not having any chest pain, she said it would be safe to take a sleeping pill. I slept until 9:30 the next morning, performed a few tasks, and went right back to bed.

I never regretted going to the wedding. But I did use the experience to help me take my enthusiasm down a notch or two.

Here's an email I received from a Healing Hearts friend in response to my comments about the fun I'd had at the wedding and the scare I'd experienced on my way home:

> Dear Linda, I read your email with awe. One line struck my heart: "I just get so high on life. I have GOT to learn to pace myself." This says it all about how you have chosen to live life, full throttle, enjoying the sheer luxury of being alive to experience the next miracle, the next smile from your grandchildren, the next celebration, the next laugh, and yes, the next challenge.
>
> One of the things I so admire and value about you is how fully and enthusiastically you witnessed and celebrated my life and my journey. I learned so much from being in your presence and watching how you dealt with the same life-and-death issues I was dealing with. I felt so defeated and hopeless when I entered the Healing Hearts program and thought I could not possibly keep up the fight.
>
> But you taught me, more than anyone else in the program, that I can choose to see my life as an adventure, be grateful for the miracle of each day, and bring the best game I have to every minute of every day. I was inspired by your irrepressible spirit, your courage, and your joy in living.

Who, me? See what I mean when I say I had amazing love and support around me? I was just being my loud, loving, goofy self, which I was finally comfortable showing. For most of my life I had felt uncomfortable in my own skin.

* * *

On November 7th I had an appointment with Dr. Hassidim, the hematologist on my transplant team. During our conversation I was reminded about the complications I had experienced during my 2004 bypass surgery. I could have another adverse reaction to Heparin, the strong blood-thinning drug. There was a point during transplantation when that drug was typically used, but I was told there was an alternate drug that could be used. The quandary was that the medical team did not like to use that drug because its effects were not reversible. The effects of Heparin could be reversed if a problem arose.

Since I'd had a problem with it before, this team would be extra-vigilant and ready with other options. In searching for more details about what had happened in 2004, the Scripps team said they were not one hundred percent sure that Heparin was the problem. Since then, I had taken a test that indicated I was not allergic to that drug. The clotting I had experienced during my bypass surgery could have been caused by some other factor. The doctor also learned that Heparin had been used on me when two stents had been inserted after my angioplasty, in May of 2006.

My appointment with the hematologist was late in the day. I was tired, and I had not brought a friend with me. So much for the positive and exciting thoughts about having a heart transplant. This was real. This was serious. This was a reasonable time for a few tears.

After our in-depth discussion, the doctor began a physical exam. He caught me totally off guard when he asked me, "Why do you even need a heart transplant?"

I'm pretty sure I blubbered, "I don't know. My cardiologists told me I need one." So much for any maturity I may have gained while taking responsibility for my own health decisions since 2005.

The first thing I heard from Dr. Jaski, the next day, was, "I got a call from Dr. Hassidim. He said he was afraid he had frazzled you." Dr. J. added some funny comments and confirmed that I did need a new heart. In the doctor's defense, he said, "He was just being very conservative. That's a good thing." Dr. J. added, "All the doctors on your team will be meeting today to put their heads and tests together. Next week Dr. Hassidim will give you a report on the meeting."

Dr. Jaski said I had a breathing and fluid-retention problem. Tiredness and an enlarged heart were other factors. He said he and Dr. Heywood had been discussing my case for a long time. They both felt that my heart would last only two to three more years. He also spent a long time telling me about the time and effort my transplant team was putting in to understand possible complications. He assured me they would be ready for anything.

Once again, I was good to go. Wait a minute, doesn't that sound like I was happy to be so sick? I was happy that my doctors knew I had a problem, and that they had a solution. My sister Jean had not had that advantage for most of her life. I can't imagine the physical and emotional pain of being very sick and not being taken seriously some of the time.

* * *

In an email I sent to my family on November 9th, I wrote,

> Vicki, my super new nurse practitioner, had told me during my last appointment that I might get a new heart soon. When I asked why, I learned that a person can accept a heart that is fifty percent smaller or a hundred fifty percent bigger than their own heart. Based on body size, a smaller person has an advantage.

"And you're a golden receiver," Vicki had added.

"What?" I did a double take on those words. "Like a dog, a Golden Retriever?"

"No, not exactly." She laughed. "A golden receiver has blood type AB positive and is able to accept any other type of blood." That gave me an even bigger advantage for finding a match. Wow!

* * *

After I announced to my evening women's group that I would soon be on the waiting list for a heart transplant, my friend Diane approached me. She asked, "Would you mind if I go with you when you go to the hospital for your surgery?"

The cell phone call or pager ring can come anytime, day or night. I'd been told I had to get to the hospital within one to two hours of receiving the call. With Craig in Singapore and Kristin in Idaho, there was no chance that either of them would be with me. I had recently envisioned the doctor coming out of the operating room after my transplant surgery, calling out, "Who is here for Linda LeVier?" The question would be followed by a deadly silence.

Since my main concern up to now had been getting approval to even be on the list, I hadn't considered asking someone to go with me for the surgery. Diane graciously accepted the task of being my family liaison. She would talk with the medical staff and then call Kristin, who would pass the information on to Craig.

What a profound relief I felt when I thanked Diane for her offer. I knew she had been a nurse before she'd had children. She said she would enjoy sharing the experience with me. I used the opportunity to invite her to come to my next appointment with the hematologist, as I had decided I could not face him alone again. When she said she could go, she gave me my second wave of relief.

The tone of this meeting was much better. Diane asked a lot of questions, using her "nurse" voice. The doctor had a softer manner as we discussed the possible complications and options. He shared information and concerns from the surgeons. I gave my consent to use Heparin for the shortest possible amount of time. Diane and I were reassured that my medical team was ready for a successful outcome after all their research and preparations.

I treated Diane to lunch with pie as we talked about the appointment and anything else that came to mind. She had been helping me deal with my feelings and emotions. Many people in my generation were taught to "keep their dirty laundry at home." Stiff upper lip. Poker face. When someone asks, "How are you?" you say "Fine"—no matter how much you could use a word of encouragement or a hug. I am glad I learned, in time, to trust the goodness in people.

In addition, I couldn't wait to start "paying forward" the kindness and help I'd been gifted.

✶ ✶ ✶

During a conversation with Marilyn D. from WomenHeart, I mentioned that I needed more chances to laugh. I said I had heard something about laughter groups on TV once. She told me she had seen some notices in a local newspaper. I soon got a call from her with contact information for a woman who offered laughing meditations. The concept did not make sense to me. Isn't meditation supposed to be quiet?

My curiosity and need for more laughter in my life led me to Sarito Sun, who was introduced to laughing meditation in the 1970s by her guru, Osho.

Over the phone, Sarito described her sessions and encouraged me to attend one at the Chopra Center, located in my city, Carlsbad. I have already written about what a hard time I have sitting still and quieting my mind for meditation. But … I wanted to laugh! What the heck, I'd been doing healthy eating, exercising, support groups, and taking my pills. Laughing couldn't hurt, could it?

I drove to the Chopra Center. I walked down the hall and entered a room decorated with tapestries and Buddha statues, its walls hung with ornate rugs. I indulged in a pervasive sarcastic thought: meditation and laughter? Really?

The people in the room were already talking and laughing with each other. There was Sarito, a grown-older San Francisco hippie flower child. She was a charming woman in a long, flowing skirt, with a full-of-joy face and twinkling eyes. Then she laughed. So we laughed. We couldn't help but join in with her infectious, lilting, giggly laugh. My sarcastic thoughts dissolved. I knew immediately I was about to have a good experience.

Sarito's "laughter is the best medicine" lecture included the statement that one of the goals of meditation is to "get you out of your head." That idea caught my attention. Though I don't remember much of what I heard that day, I do remember the sound of the laughter, the variety of laughs, and how hard it was to stop laughing.

Sarito was not a comedian, but she was funny. Soon all of us were funny, in our actions. No one told jokes. We just allowed ourselves to laugh, simply because the act of laughing felt good. We ended the session by lying on our backs, breathing quietly and deeply.

Driving home, I thought about how I felt. I was a bit surprised to realize I felt calm, a decidedly foreign feeling for me. But then I sensed tiny explosions, similar to those I've felt when tasting the candy they call Pop Rocks, going off in my tummy and chest. Calm and tingly. Not the scary tingling I'd felt in my left arm on many occasions. Calm and sparkly. I knew I wanted to attend more laughing meditation sessions.

The best part was that the calm lasted for a long time. I'd gone in with the painful pressure in my abdomen I felt most of the time in those days, but I experienced none of that during the session or for hours afterward. I slept well that night.

Sarito did not host weekly meetings, but I did go to laugh with her whenever I could.

✶ ✶ ✶

At the next WomenHeart meeting, someone suggested we name our hearts. The idea was to give them an identity we could visualize and address with positive messages. One woman encouraged me to name the new heart that would be coming to me. We laughed at the silly ideas.

At home I thought about names for my new heart, just as most pregnant women consider names for their babies before the birth. I visualized my new heart, then abandoned the vision when I got a pang of concern for my birth heart. That heart needed my love to keep it as strong as possible. I quickly came up with its name, "My Loyal and Courageous Heart," and I visualized my heart that had been working so hard, even though it was badly damaged, before the 2004 angiogram had revealed its condition. "Hang in there, My Loyal and Courageous Heart. We are getting ready to find a replacement so that you can get a well-deserved rest!"

I also gave a name to the heart I hoped to receive: "Gift from the Universe."

20
Scariest Thoughts

Quiet days were in order as I prepared for a special celebration. I had been told that the way was cleared for me to be put on the waiting list. November 19th was to be my first day, but I had one more medication to take for a bit longer. Nevertheless, it was time for my Heart Transplant Kick-Off party!

I laid a red paper carpet on the path to my front door for my guests. Sherin provided fresh flowers. We had the traditional buffet potluck, with lots of yummies and sparkling juice in the fridge. My crazy condo neighbors came, plus a few other close friends. Cindy (my recent massage therapist), Diane, and a couple who had been "adopted" by our condo group arrived. (Cindy had also offered to go to the hospital with me. She would be Diane's backup.)

My favorite memory of that party is a dictate that came from Diane. She looked into the eyes of each guest in turn as she said emphatically, "Do NOT let Linda drive herself to the hospital when she gets the call that there is a heart available for her!!!" By the end of the party, I had everyone's home and cell phone numbers in my cell phone.

My home was alive with happy energy. Yes, the reason for the celebration was sobering, but the mood was upbeat. Honestly, I contend that I never heard a negative word from any person while I eagerly awaited the event I hoped would extend my life. Every day I seemed to meet new people who chose to look for the good that surrounds us.

My next appointment with Dr. Jaski was on Tuesday, November 21st. When Vicki came into the examining room, I asked whether she had any idea when I would be put on the list. "Today," she announced as she handed me the official letter required by UNOS (United Network for Organ Sharing). Its purpose was to notify all patients, in writing, of the outcome of their evaluation.

I read, "You were presented on November 21, 2006, to the Heart Transplant Selection Committee and were accepted as a candidate." The next paragraph confirmed that my name had been placed on the waiting list that very day for a heart transplant, to be performed at Sharp Memorial Hospital.

I don't remember anything else about the appointment, other than thanking Vicki, Dr. Jaski, and Kathy, the front-desk go-to gal. As the years passed, Kathy seemed more like a friend than a staff person whenever I called with a question.

Now I can admit that my scariest thoughts had started when I learned I needed a heart transplant, and continued until the time Vicki assured me I was truly on the waiting list. The official letter she handed me, with the backing of UNOS, cinched the deal. I felt a strong sense of comfort that I had the best possible safety net under me.

A few weeks earlier, soon after a heart transplant became a possibility, a friend had said, "Oh, I've never known anyone with a heart transplant." I had countered with, "Oh, neither have I!"

I wanted a way to connect with friends and relatives as my heart adventure unfolded. Having few computer skills, I struggled with setting up a group email list. The phrase "New Heart Adventure" was my choice for the email subject box.

Working on the emails created a good distraction from what my body was experiencing. I also had to work out a way for Kristin to continue to send the emails when I was in the hospital. Being ill was a full-time occupation!

One unique email was sent to group members from someone who called himself "ssk" (no full name given). He began with a plea to the others that they be as candid as he in sharing how we had met:

> I had arrived in Casablanca for R&R. It was 1942, and my commanding officer told me … I needed a break … I walked into the bar … the air was thick with sweet-smelling smoke … My lungs were doing the hula … I hear this singing … her name was Linda … Linda Majestic … she slides over to the bar … looking sideways at me, she smirked. "Another soldier boy looking for mommy," she growled … "What kinda name is Majestic?" I growled back … It's LeVier, sweetie, Linda

> LeVier … never could get that song she sang
> outta my head … A million years later, and
> a lotta hurtin' in between, I land in Carls-
> bad … My downstairs neighbor gives me the
> scoop on the rest of the people in the joint …
> she mentions a Linda LeVier … WHAT!!!!!!
> … yes, Linda left Morocco eighteen years
> ago after hangin' up her singin' career …
> Who'da thunk it?

I got the funniest responses from other readers. Just for the record, I was two years old in 1942 and doing my singing in New York, probably in diapers.

By the way, that email came from Sherin, decidedly the craziest of my crazy condo neighbors. My friends were completely aware of my declining health, but they kept me amused. No one treated me gingerly unless I put out a signal that I could use some TLC.

✷ ✷ ✷

Thanksgiving was set to be a quiet day until I received an invitation to join Cathleen and Jeff's extended family. The gathering was casual and friendly. My slow walking took them back to Cathleen's condition of the year before. I benefitted from seeing Cathleen handling her lively ten-month-old son. Her dramatic increase in wellness gave me hope for my future. I remember Omana telling me, "Linda, you don't remember how good health feels."

The Sharp Heart Transplant Support Group holiday party on December 7th was quite an event. I drove myself, in heavy commuter traffic, and arrived a little late. The large room was packed with people talking, laughing, and eating. I had to ask, "Am I at the right party?" because the table was overloaded with pizza, fried chicken, pasta dishes, creamed vegetables, and more. I put on my plate the healthiest items I could find, but I really wanted a piece or two of the pizza.

Just before we gathered for the white-elephant gift exchange, a man tapped me on my shoulder. He had overheard me talking to another guest. He'd received his heart transplant two years earlier, and wanted to assure me I would be fine. I told him I had been reading about the possible side effects of the drugs I would be taking. He said he hadn't had any side effects, and then gave me a warm hug.

Each December now, I happily display a snowman mug with a stirring stick for hot chocolate. I took it from someone during the white-elephant gift exchange. On the bottom of the mug I wrote the date of the party. That was my first holiday party with the heart transplant community.

✶ ✶ ✶

During my cardiology appointment on the 11th, the first person I saw was Kristi, Dr. Jaski's other nurse practitioner. In came a burst of sunshine with a playful smile. This journey just kept getting better. I rattled off my questions and some stories. She laughed and said, "We have looked at your tests very carefully. We know you are in need of a new heart. You just look so healthy and have so much good spirit!"

Again I heard I might get a new heart by Christmas. I'm a little embarrassed to admit that I thought, and maybe said out loud, "I love Christmas. Do you think we could wait until it's over?" Didn't I realize how sick I was? I know I felt safer and, I guess, healthier knowing that help was available if I felt real distress.

What I did not say out loud was that 2007 would soon be here. I love sevens. My birthday is July 7th. Wouldn't it be perfect if I received a new heart in 2007? Please don't be too hard on me. This was a weird time in my life. Anytime my mind got still, it charged off in wild directions that caused me to laugh inside.

✶ ✶ ✶

Ruthann, a condo neighbor, surprised me with a most appropriate and meaningful gift. I opened the box and saw a charming ceramic angel in muted colors. She had soft brown hair and brown wire-loop wings. In her hands she held a red heart. Ruthann told me the angel was holding and protecting the heart I would get. I was to go on taking care of myself. The angel would release my heart when the time was right.

I was deeply touched. I placed the angel in a prominent place, where I would see her often. Sitting alone and gazing at her, I decided she was the embodiment of Allison Michelle, the baby I'd lost to an ectopic pregnancy. I believe Allison had been in the hospital at the time of my bypass surgery, speaking the names of two nurses. Now I could see her, too. And I felt her presence.

A few days later, a second angel flew in from Santa Fe, New Mexico. My college friend Ann told me she had seen the angel and just had to buy it for me. This metal angel was in a flying position, with her arms bent so her hands were over her heart. On an edge of her gown were the words, "Protect this woman."

156

I chose to think of this angel as my sister Jean. I found a perfect spot on the headboard of my bed where I could place her using the attached purple ribbon.

During my heart sojourn I received several hearts and angels in various forms. I knew I had a big support team, and the tangible treasures and thoughtfully written emails strengthened my spirit and courage.

The following is an email received by members of my New Heart Adventure email group on December 17th:

> Hello, friends and family of Linda,
>
> Many of you (and I think of Linda's son and daughter especially) are keeping up with how Linda is faring based on her emails. I thought you might be interested in a first-hand-witness account of how Linda is doing, from someone else.
>
> I am Linda's friend and neighbor. I see and talk to Linda fairly regularly. Last evening, we both were in attendance at an Open House held by another neighbor of ours. I can tell you with assurance that Linda looked fine (wonderful, actually, in her festive outfit) and was in wonderful spirits and form.
>
> She was (as you would expect) the life of the party. She was the first one there and one of the last ones to leave and kept everyone laughing the whole time. While there is no question that Linda faces a very serious medical threat with a major procedure ahead of her, she absolutely does what she needs to do to stay as healthy and strong as possible and has a positive attitude and spirit like no one else I have ever known.
>
> So, for those of you who don't get to see Linda on a regular basis, know that what she says in her emails is true. (Last night's party was evidence of that.)
>
> JoAnn

✳ ✳ ✳

In late December a loud, grinding sound came from my refrigerator. I called a repair service and described the problem. The person on the phone said it was probably the generator. I was prepared for an expensive house call. Yes, indeed, the repairman gave me the bad news. He went to his truck to get the replacement generator and set to work.

As he got ready to pull out the old motor, he said, "It's an easy operation, a lot like a heart transplant. I just make four cuts to the holding wires, pull out the motor, put in the new one, and connect the four wires."

"Really? It's funny you should use that analogy. I am now on the Heart Transplant Waiting List."

I imagine he has told that story as often as I have.

✶ ✶ ✶

I decided I did not want my sister Marilyn to be with me during the holidays. Since I was now on the waiting list, I didn't want the possibility of getting The Call that a heart was available while she was here. She would be stuck in my condo while I was in the hospital for two weeks. Craig's family was still in Singapore. She would be better off enjoying the holidays with my nephew's family in San Francisco.

I did want to put up my favorite Christmas decorations. At my Kick-Off party, several friends offered to help me. In came the crew, with Sherin, the big boss, barking, "Come on, faster, faster. We're on the clock. Look how many decorations she has. We should have known!"

Sue offered to prepare Christmas dinner for me if she and her parents could celebrate with me in my beautifully decorated home. She had been in on the decorating. I quickly agreed, on the condition that she and her parents consider singing Christmas carols with me. What a deal! That was an offer none of us could refuse.

Sue did a lot of work before they arrived. My home was filled with the mouth-watering smells of the final preparations. Sue's mother and father also had medical issues, which had led to healthy recipe choices. I can still remember how my taste buds fired up with each bite of Maryland crab cakes, asparagus, brown and wild rice, and sourdough bread. Chef Linda added some veggie finger foods. The sparkling cider was a festive touch, but the key lime pie took the meal over the top!

The dinner conversation was livelier than either Sue or I could have predicted. I began by asking Sue's father about his World War II experiences. He took the bait and entertained us with facts and personal anecdotes. Everyone has stories. I am getting better at encouraging people to share theirs with me. Our memorable evening ended with singing Christmas carols, just as I had hoped would happen.

2006 came to an end with a New Year's Eve party at my home. JoAnn, Diane, Ruthann, Sue, and I let go of that year together, wishing each other good health and happiness in 2007. As we made a midnight toast with our bubbly apple-cranberry drink, I got teary. Turning to JoAnn, I said, "Here we go!"

Strong, meaningful hugs from each of my gal pals boosted my courage to face 2007. I had the feeling an exciting challenge was just around the corner.

My roller coaster highs and lows had been about even in 2006. The concern about my physical health was balanced by my confidence in my medical teams from two hospitals. Any emotional low spots were overshadowed by the strong friendship bonds I was developing as I added new friends to those I already had.

* * *

The light tone of my writing is true to my public self. A majority of my time alone was also upbeat, but maybe not as boisterous. I haven't started to talk out loud to myself, but I have a running dialogue going on in my head. I'm getting better at laughing out loud at minor funny things that happen wherever I am. I am grateful to my Healing Hearts friends, WomenHeart members, Dr. Heywood, and Sarito for reminding me that the act of laughing is medicinal. I don't have to wait for the big knee-slappers. I can easily start to laugh out loud when I think of something that made me laugh in the past.

I am a thoughtful and sometimes overly serious person. So far, I have not commented on my thoughts about the heart I was waiting to receive. The circle of life includes life and death. It is hard to accept the fact that someone has to die before a healthy heart becomes available to be transplanted to another person.

Tranquilizers and antidepressants are frequently needed by survivors of an illness or accident. If friends are in an accident and just one survives, the survivor may find himself dealing with gratitude and remorse at the same time. I don't have any words that have not been said by clergy and philosophers. I did understand that a person would die sometime without my knowledge. If that person agreed to be an organ donor, as I had, then his or her heart might come to me.

One way I could help my doctors was to acknowledge the sad realities that accompanied my condition and the possible solutions. It was important and healthy for me to do what I could to keep my stress level low. Accepting the help of my friends was my pleasure and, I believe, my responsibility.

Come on, 2007! I was ready and willing to handle whatever might be thrown my way.

21

Anticipation Jitters

I had invited Diane to spend the night because I didn't want her to drive home on New Year's Eve. We decided to begin 2007 with a walk on the beach. When we got to a certain point, Diane recalled the time she'd seen a man "drawing" a labyrinth in the sand. He'd used tools of his own making to create a network of paths on which people could walk and perhaps enjoy a spiritual experience.

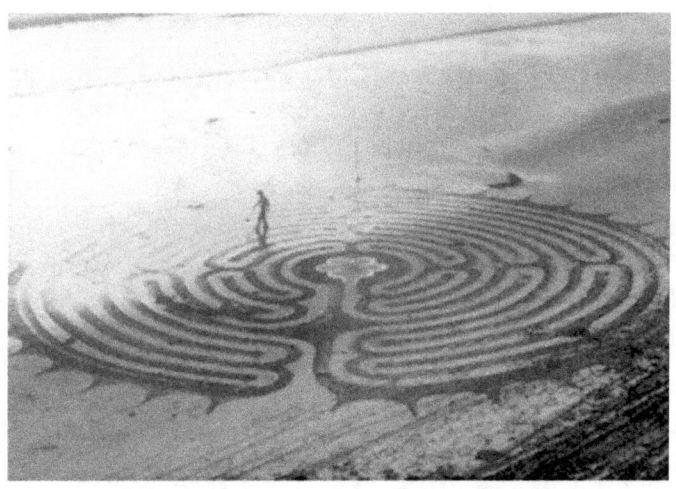

Kirkos working on his labyrinth on the beach—
a soulful gift for anyone to walk before the tide rolls in

All of a sudden she said, "There are his tools. He must be around here." He came into view, and we had a long talk. After giving us warm hugs, he handed me his business card. I dropped it into the bag that held my pager. Meeting Kirkos (his artist name) felt like a good omen for this new year.

✴ ✴ ✴

The next day Craig was back from Singapore again, but we had only a little time together. We were able to get an appointment with Dr. Jaski, who gave Craig a review of my current condition: United Network of Organ Sharing (UNOS) Status 2, with advanced ischemic cardiomyopathy. Craig already knew about my continuing problem with fluid retention and pressure in the chest. He had a chance to ask about the transplant procedure and when he should return to the states after my surgery. I felt better knowing Craig had met my new doctor and had his questions answered.

* * *

UNOS Wait List Statuses for Heart Transplantation

Status 1A — These patients are at the top of the waiting list. They usually include patients in the intensive care unit who are on life support and/or high-dose intravenous (IV) medications to support their heart function, or who have a ventricular assist device (VAD) or extracorporeal membrane oxygenation (ECMO) to support their heart function.

Status 1B — These patients have end-stage heart failure and are at home on a ventricular assist device (VAD) or continuous IV heart medication (inotrope medication) that makes the heart beat stronger.

Status 2 — These patients do not meet the criteria for Status 1A or 1B. Most often, these patients are waiting at home for a donor heart and are taking oral heart failure medication.

* * *

A few days later, I shared with Craig a dream I'd had the night before. In the dream I was in a mall, and a stranger pushed me down and pinned me to the ground. At the top of my lungs I yelled, "Yes! I do need a new heart, Dr. Heywood!" I'm sure that was the first time I had acknowledged to myself that I was indeed very sick.

* * *

Just before Craig left, he presented me with a huge poster bearing two photos. One was of his two girls in hot-weather Singapore clothes, and the other showed Kristin's children in cold-weather Idaho clothes. I was to take the poster with me to the hospital when I got "The Call." Do you remember the poster I had in my ICU room in 2004, with photos of my three grandchildren? Petra had since joined the family, and this new "We love you Grandma" inspirational poster included her. Kristin and Craig knew I would get extra pleasure looking at it during my wait.

Another photo treasure came by email from Kirkos—two beautiful photos of a labyrinth he had created. I gave one to Diane and framed the other for myself. I still have it in a place where I see it often. The sight of it makes me smile and remember the good times I enjoyed during my medical roller coaster ride.

After Craig's talk with Dr. Jaski, I thought that Kristin might benefit from talking with Vicki, NP, by phone. They had a good conversation. Kristin was able to get her questions answered. I'm sure Vicki did her reassuring magic to help Kristin understand what was ahead.

I attended a Laughter Happy Hour at the Encinitas Cancer Center the day before my January 11th appointment with Dr. Heywood. When the good doctor came in and saw how healthy I looked, he said, "Linda, you are consistently inconsistent!" I'd heard that before. We talked about a possible trip to Idaho to visit Kristin's family.

I brought up the subject of the trip to Idaho with Dr. Jaski on the 16th. He gave me permission to go. As for the transplant waiting list, I would be placed "on hold" the day I left, and put back on when I returned home.

The idea sounded good until Nurse Practitioner Vicki told me that two hearts had become available that were possibilities for me. Although they went to people who were more in need, this information helped me decide not to take the trip.

The rest of January brought me movies at home with friends, long walks near the beach, crazy laughter on Belly Laugh Day, a massage, a hair appointment, a Condo Crazies' brunch, and another echocardiogram. My latest EF result was 25%—higher than some of my previous scores. My good old heart was doing its best for me.

Just before the end of January, Sue let me borrow a movie she was sure I would enjoy. I didn't pay attention to what it was about, didn't read the blurb on the box. Thank goodness I was alone during the viewing. It turned out to be a sweet story about a widower and a woman he'd met. As the movie progressed, I realized that the plot involved a heart transplant.

I shed a few tears, and then began to sob. It was my first big-time stress-releasing cry since the onset of my heart problems. Crying can be cathartic.

(The movie really was a romantic comedy, not a heavy piece of work. If you have not already seen *Return to Me*, you might enjoy watching it.)

In February, I received emails from friends who had picked "the day" when I would get my new heart. I put all their guesses (or wishes) on a desk calendar. Some of them were upset when it turned out that their day was not the big day for me. I let them choose a second date, of course, to add to my calendar.

Not everyone was comfortable with my light-hearted game. (Did anyone guess the exact date of my surgery? Read on to find out.)

Then there was the email from a friend who thought I'd written that I'd laughed with a group "in the buff." She reread my email, which said that our group had laughed on the bluff overlooking the Pacific Ocean. That laughter group had been led by Gaga, a woman I'd met at one of Sarito's events. Gaga offered free laughter sessions once a week at the South Ponto Beach bluff in Carlsbad. How I looked forward to Mondays at 3:30pm!

Gaga's laughter sessions were called "Laughter Yoga," while Sarito titled her sessions "Laughing Meditation." Both women had been recently certified as laughter leaders by Dr. Madan Kataria, the founder of Laughter Yoga. He believed that the act of laughing was such a healthy activity that it should not be reserved for a good joke or a funny event. He had developed a set of "exercises" that helped participants laugh by choice, without benefit of a humorous igniter. For most people, the induced laughter was contagious enough to lead to genuine full-of-fun laughter.

Craig was back in town again. On the drive from the airport I played a section of the CD Sarito had recorded. The first part had her opening remarks about the physical and emotional benefits of adding extra laughing to your life. Track eight was all laughing, recorded during one of the free-for-all laughter sessions with participants lying on their backs.

On my way to medical appointments I often started the CD on track eight. I'd tell myself I didn't feel like laughing, but I would listen. Within minutes, I would join the laughers as I maneuvered through the traffic. I was often asked why I looked so happy when I arrived at the office. Duh.

My activities that month were low-key, with phone calls, walks, a HeartScarves exhibit at the library, tax preparation meetings, day and evening social/support groups, and an evening of fun with the Condo Crazies playing Mexican Train, a domino game.

* * *

My weight had risen to one hundred twenty-four pounds, but there had been no change in my heart condition. Once again I was considering the trip to Idaho. Dr. Jaski said the trip might be good medicine for me. I booked a flight and was to be ready for the airport shuttle at 4:30 on Tuesday morning, February 20th.

Later that day, in Idaho, I had a hard time walking the uneven terrain of a park, the site of an annual fair. Back indoors, it was good to be able to hold Aengus and Petra and talk with Kristin and Brian. It was undeniably therapeutic for me to have face time with my daughter, if just for a short while. We had two full days before I flew home on Friday, the 23rd.

✶ ✶ ✶

By the 24th, I was exhausted, bloated, and teary. Our condos had been painted. Thank goodness my ever-so-special condo friends had helped with removing and then replacing the plants and furniture on my front deck.

I ended the month with daily ups and downs. A massage, a manicure, and the laughter group helped lift my spirits, but I had no stamina. I was beginning to feel lousy, but I continued my walks.

The first day of March, I had a good walk and then a visit with Sue and Janette, my condo neighbors. Uh oh. I stayed up too late. The next day started out fine, with a haircut and a facial, but by 4:30 that afternoon I was wiped out and teary again. So much stomach and chest pressure! I had hoped to go Sufi dancing that evening.

At my appointment with Dr. Jaski, I told him I wasn't able to sleep at night and that I felt hungry but could only tolerate ice water or yogurt. He adjusted some of my meds.

By March 7th, I had begun to turn down social invitations. No more night meetings.

Stop! Enough of that.

✶ ✶ ✶

I bought myself flowers. What the heck. I decided to attend the evening women's circle. I was hurting, so I thought I would stay just a short time. I made it through the whole meeting, but I think I sank into a soft chair, looking like a pregnant woman who was way overdue. However, I felt so good by the end of the meeting that I bought a spicy, greasy beef-and-cheese taco on the way home … and it tasted delicioso!

On March 9th, I met a new neighbor and her little girl. After she heard about my condition, she took on the role of caretaker. Over the next couple of days she brought me soothing Chinese dishes that I thoroughly enjoyed and appreciated. I didn't want to take advantage of my illness. I was overwhelmed with gratitude for the support, gifts, and offers to help me. Yes, happy tears came easily, too.

A WomenHeart meeting with a HeartMath session was a good distraction before getting another echocardiogram.

* * *

Vicki called and said I had an ejection fraction result of 40%, way up from my January result of 25%. I'd thought that EF results were not known to bobble around. Vicki also commented that I was dehydrated. Where was the fluid going? "You need to stop taking the booster diuretic," she said.

"… But I can't handle the weight gain!"

"Okay. Try one-fourth tablet." She decided I needed to see Dr. Pressman, a gastroenterologist within the Sharp Hospital system.

I was able to see Dr. Pressman the next day. I liked him immediately. When he stepped into the room to see me, he asked whether he could take care of another patient first. He said he wanted to have more time to go over my condition with me.

"No problem. I have a book," I said.

After a good discussion with me, he pulled a few strings to quickly line up several tests, including a colonoscopy.

The Sharp medical staff had to be sure there were no GI issues. I shared my news with a few people. Craig and my friend Ron both responded immediately with great concern. They told me to be sure Dr. Pressman was aware of the bleeding problems I'd had in 2004. Craig told me to show the doctor certain pages and paragraphs from his notes.

Based on my experience with heavy bleeding in 2004, Craig thought a colonoscopy before the transplant sounded scarier than the heart transplant surgery. We knew that the previous problem had been due to the blood-thinning drugs, but Craig was concerned about my fragile GI area. But he understood that the colonoscopy should be done if other less invasive tests didn't provide enough information.

Dr. Pressman looked at Craig's notes, and took time to discuss with me the need for the colonoscopy. Then he said, "I'm afraid they will not let you have the heart transplant if you don't have the colonoscopy first." I told him I understood the situation and gave my consent.

On March 19th I had a CT scan in which no problems were found.

I had been instructed not to drive on March 20th, the day of the colonoscopy. Friends came to my rescue. Condo neighbors Chuck and Anita said they'd leave me off and then have a "day date" for themselves before returning to take me home. They made it easier for me to accept their help by sharing how they would benefit from helping me.

I had fun with Chuck and Anita on the drive to Sharp Memorial Hospital. Due to my nervousness, I'd slept very little the night before. They did an excellent job of lifting my spirits. The day daters left me off with big smiles and a "See ya later."

My nerves were scrambled when I donned my gown and climbed up onto the operating table. As soon as I saw Dr. Pressman, I felt better. I shared a secret with him. I told him I had experienced a "sign" in the middle of the night, right after I was put on the official waiting-for-a-heart-transplant list. I'd felt a calming message that there would be no heart transplant complications. Considering the complicated circumstances of my 2004 bypass surgery, the "sign" had made a big impression on me.

"Do you think that reassuring message would include the colonoscopy?" I asked.

He appeared to take my words seriously. He put one hand to his chin, using the other hand to prop up the opposite arm at the elbow, much like Rodin's statue *The Thinker*. After a brief pause he said, "I think it's a total package."

That sweet and funny memory continues to be one of my favorites.

When I woke up after the colonoscopy, the nurse at my side said everything had gone well. They hadn't found any problems. Then she added, "Dr. Pressman wanted me to tell you that there was not one drop of blood during the procedure!"

The next day, I learned that Dr. Pressman had seen a nodule on my lung that should not be a problem. The CT stomach scan and the colonoscopy results were good, yet the feeling of extreme tightness persisted in my torso.

I told Dr. Heywood on March 22nd that the pressure felt like I was wearing an old-fashioned corset, the kind you see in the movies with a maid pulling corset strings with all her might to make the lady's waist tiny. My weight was at one hundred twenty-six, far over the hundred-eighteen outer limit set by my medical team. (I'm only five feet one inch tall.)

Dr. Heywood wanted me to check into Scripps Green Hospital. I declined his recommendation, saying I should probably go to Sharp Memorial Hospital since I was now on their heart-transplant waiting list. At this point I was seeing Dr. Jaski, the cardiologist at Sharp Memorial Hospital, where I would have my heart transplant surgery. I also remained under the care of my congestive heart failure cardiologist, who was with the Scripps medical system.

My favorite excerpts from Dr. Heywood's notes, March 22, 2007:

> Weight has gone up; appetite is less; liver is mildly enlarged; fluid overloaded. She is an alert and somewhat tearful female, much less animated than usual; she needs to get off nine pounds of water.

> I discussed admission to the hospital, but she has refused this; I would like to get labs today, but she requested not to go to the lab because recent blood draws and IVs have left her feeling a bit like a pincushion.

I remember feeling like an overdue pregnant elephant as I lumbered across the parking lot. Just as I arrived at my car, my cell phone rang. It was Vicki, NP, telling me to drive straight to Sharp Memorial Hospital. "May I get some lunch on the way?" I asked. She said I could have a very small amount of food.

That was the day that I learned that some sandwich places sell a three-inch sandwich in addition to their advertised six- and twelve-inch sandwiches. It tasted good. Do you see the pattern? As soon as I am sure I am being monitored, I start to feel better. With all of the bloating, I either didn't want to eat or was afraid to eat. Now that I was heading to the safety net of a hospital, I knew I could handle eating something.

Several times on my good days, when I didn't look or feel sick, I said, "Please, don't take me off the Waiting List!" I was convinced I needed a new heart. I didn't want my good days to confuse my doctors into thinking I was getting healthier on my own.

I learned that I would be staying at Sharp Memorial Hospital for five days so that I could be watched and tested in a new-to-me way. I was given a powerful intravenous dose of medicine to strengthen my heart. Then the medicine was stopped, to see how quickly my heart would lose strength. The data from that test showed that I needed a 24/7 intravenous stream of the medicine.

From then on, I would receive Milrinone—a short-term treatment for life-threatening heart failure—around the clock, via an IV connecting me to a bag that held the medicine. That moved my need-for-a-new-heart status from Level 2 to the 1-B level.

On March 27th, wearing a hospital gown over my own long pants, I drove the three freeways that would take me home. The contraption I had to wear looked like a shaving kit with a shoulder strap. The gizmo was too big to go through the sleeve of the sweatshirt I had worn to the hospital—thus the hospital gown. Thank goodness I had no need to stop to pick up a new prescription.

A home nurse was scheduled to visit me the next day to explain how to change the medicine bottles and batteries in the medical bag. Remember, I lived alone. Okay, I said to myself, we're getting serious now. This is a bit scary.

I had to learn how to sleep cuddled up to a lifesaving bag.

I know I had a worried look on my face when the pleasant nurse arrived the next day to educate me on my new routine. I was smart to have asked my neighbor Ruthann to be with me as I heard this new information.

The nurse reassured me that she would come regularly until I convinced her I was comfortable making the changes by myself. I warned her that she might have to keep coming until I got a new heart—and who knew how long that would be? She came again the next day. Sue and Anita were my extra eyes and ears and moral support during that visit.

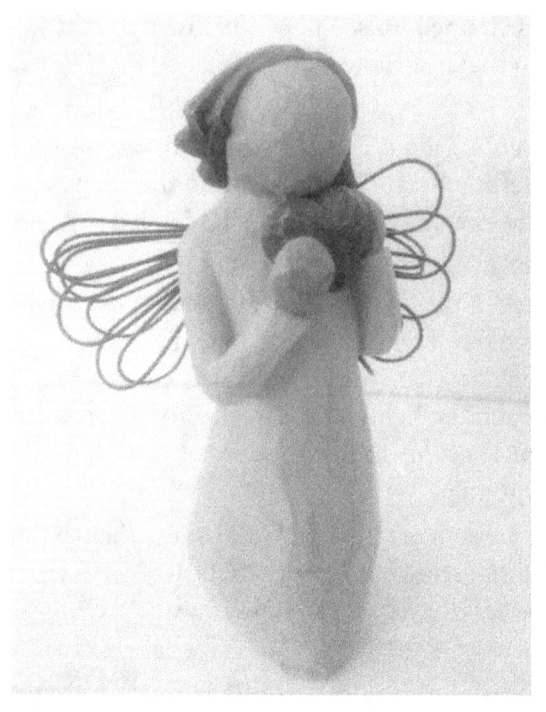

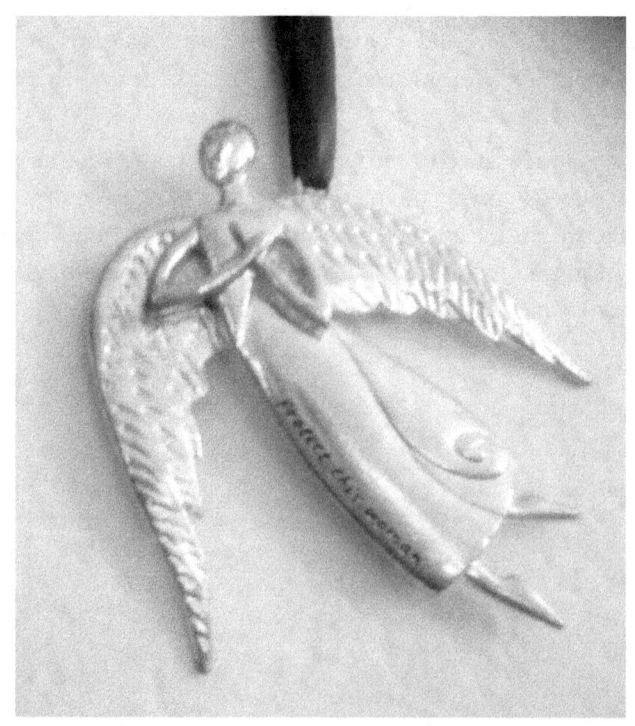

22

Patio Party

Gradually I grew accustomed to my new appendage. Dressing each day was a challenge, as I had to find clothes with sleeves wide enough to allow the bag to pass through. I don't remember much about this phase, but I can still picture the little medicine bottles in my refrigerator.

It had been a while since the last brunch with my condo neighbors. Sherin proposed we consider the next Saturday, March 31st. Email invitations were sent. Some people had conflicting plans and others changed their "yes" RSVP to a "no." For the first time, I declined. I just did not feel up to going to a restaurant.

I told Sherin that JoAnn would be disappointed if we didn't get together. We would both miss being with our lively and funny friends. Without hesitation, Sherin decided he would get take-out food so that he, JoAnn, and I could eat on my front deck. I still wasn't sure I was up to the occasion, but I agreed in order to be with my two good pals.

During the last days of March, my fluid buildup was unmanageable. I was in a lot of pain, and fear was sneaking in. One night I walked over to the little angel that held a red heart. Ruthann had told me the angel was holding my new heart and knew when I would get it. I touched the angel's skirt and said out loud, "I know you know when I will get my new heart." Tearfully, I added, "Could it be soon?"

I walked to my bed and touched the metal angel, given to me by Ann. I had decided that angel represented my older sister, who had almost agreed to experimental heart-transplant surgery in 1968. As I touched the skirt, I said, "Okay, Jean, help me get through this."

The next morning, March 31st, I did my best to get into a party mood. Sherin and JoAnn would soon be with me, indulging in our Italian lunch. The "what can I wear?" predicament arose. This was by no means a formal affair, but I wanted to look reasonably festive even though I didn't feel festive inside. It was a little chilly outside, so I wore long, comfortable red velour pants, a bright yellow top, and a red jacket with sleeves wide enough for my medical bag to slip through. I was dressed to party. My mood immediately shot up!

There I was in my jazzy red outfit, ready to snack on delicious forbidden heart-disease fare. This was shaping up to be a special occasion. I even brought out my camera, which was reserved for visits with my grandchildren.

Soon after JoAnn came, Sherin arrived with the lunch. On a low-salt, low-fat diet due to my heart condition, I had planned to eat just a bit of the salad and its yummy, rich dressing. Yes, I tasted it right away. The garlic bread sat in view, tempting me to take a bite.

Before the scrumptious lasagna was added to my plate, my phone rang. I jumped up, opened the patio's sliding door, and grabbed the receiver. "What? The transplant office? What?" Stepping out to the patio, I screamed, "This is THE CALL! They have a heart for me!" I could barely stay focused enough to hear that I needed to be at Sharp Memorial Hospital within an hour and a half. Oh, my gosh!

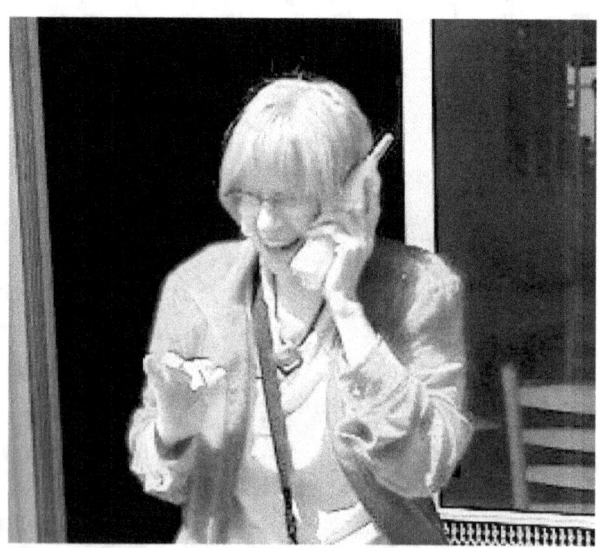

Yes, I received "The Call" the morning after I asked the ceramic angel, "Could it be soon?"

I didn't realize until much later that JoAnn had picked up my camera

172

and captured that very special moment. There I was in the photo with my bright red jacket and pants, the black medicine bag over my shoulder, waving my hands in excited gestures.

The scene quickly shifted to comical "I Love Lucy" TV craziness. Remember the episode in which Lucy and Desi get ready to go to the hospital for the birth of their baby? The three of us zigged and zagged as we handled different tasks. JoAnn picked up the food and put it in my refrigerator. Sherin began searching through my papers to find the phone number for the visiting nurse, who would soon be driving to my home. I didn't want her to wade through the San Diego freeway traffic, on a Saturday no less, only to have no one answer my doorbell.

I had to call Diane, my good friend who had offered to go to the hospital and stay with me throughout the surgery. The medical staff would communicate with her, knowing she would call my daughter, who would then call my son.

I left JoAnn and Sherin to do whatever they felt they had to do while I went upstairs to call Kristin before I sat down at my computer.

"Where are you going?" shouted Sherin.

"I have to send a message to my New Heart Adventure friends to tell them I'm going to the hospital to get my new heart."

I did warn everyone that this could be just a dry run. At any point, a mismatch could stop the surgery. Until my surgeon and his team agreed that the "new" heart was healthy and a good match for me, the transplant would not take place.

More minutes passed, and Sherin started yelling at me again. "Where are you now? What don't you understand about the need to get you to the hospital right away?"

"I have to put on my purple socks." One pair of purple socks was in my hospital bag. I'd worn that pair, by mistake, during my transplant evaluation testing. After washing them, I had put them into my hospital bag in hopes of wearing them in the OR during my surgery. I wanted to wear my other pair of purple socks on the drive to the hospital.

At long last, we were cruising down the coast highway to avoid the weekend freeway traffic. All of a sudden it hit me: A few weeks earlier I had thought, "Wouldn't it be great if Sherin could drive me to the hospital and JoAnn could sit with me in the back seat?" The likelihood of that happening had been nil, since both Sherin and JoAnn were gone all week and very busy on the weekends.

I had known that JoAnn would want to be with me. We had grown close over the last two years. But she would have been way too nervous to be my driver.

Well, there we were. Sherin maneuvered confidently through traffic while JoAnn and I sat in the back seat, stunned. I can't remember, but I assume I was chattering nervously. In spite of all the excitement, I'd remembered to bring the three-foot-by-four-foot poster bearing the photos of my four grandchildren.

Diane was already at Sharp Memorial Hospital by the time we arrived. Her first task was to find a wheelchair for me.

My last memory of Sherin is of him telling the nurse or hospital volunteer, who was about to wheel me away, "This stays with her!" He was referring to the huge poster. My memory recorded the nurse carrying the poster with the photo of my grandchildren and the endearing words. Now that I think back, Diane probably carried the poster as a hospital volunteer wheeled me to my pre-op room.

JoAnn captured another view of those last minutes. As I was wheeled into the elevator, she took a photo of me with my arms up high in a "Very good, very good, yea!" Laughter Yoga cheer. Off Diane and I went, with a wave and a quick goodbye to JoAnn and Sherin. There were no emotional words or hugs. It didn't occur to me that I might never see them again.

When the elevator door closed, JoAnn and Sherin looked at each other and one of them said, "This is big!"

23

LINDA, Welcome to 7 North!

As I write about my Sharp Memorial Hospital experience, I draw on my memories and Diane's notes. She took seriously her role of family liaison. After the surgery, she gave me a shiny red folder with a zillion hearts on the cover. Inside was her detailed account of the facts and impressions of my hospital experience, printed on lavender paper!

Diane's notes included personal reflections back to her nursing days. She met my need to keep my family informed, and she gave me so much more. Diane's notebook is a rare treasure. Her link between my medical team and my family proved invaluable.

At 2:45 that afternoon, Diane and I were taken to my pre-op room on the seventh floor. The first thing I noticed was a note in big letters on the white message board: "LINDA, Welcome to 7 North!"

> *Diane's Words*
>
> *Linda is admitted to 7th floor ... the excitement is palpable! I find it interesting. I realize that any transplant surgery would be a huge concern ... and monumental from a personal standpoint, especially after she had such fragile health for so long ... waiting, worrying, and what-if-ing like crazy. But I see firsthand how this is still a huge clinical event, too. The cardiac team is so "ticking" with excitement, yet they are so reassuring, doing everything to help Linda be comfortable and informed before each step occurs.*

My IV medical pump had run down, so the first concern was to give me the medicine I would have taken at home. We were told that the donor's heart was a perfect match for blood type and size, but that further lab work was needed. The results would not be known until about 6:00 that evening.

I was able to call Kristin to assure her that all was well, even though there would be a delay. Diane and I passed the time telling stories, laughing, and reflecting on our times together. When there was still no news at 6:00 or 7:00, Nurse Practitioner Kristi came in to tell us what to expect, time-wise, based on a typical surgical scenario.

By 7:35pm, passing the time was getting harder and we were getting sillier. We wondered whether we should call my condo friends to come and play Mexican Train dominoes with us.

I was told to remove my jewelry—the beautiful beaded bracelet made for me by Kelley, a friend from the evening women's group. I encouraged Diane to wear it. I learned later from Diane that she had felt a strong spiritual energy connection with me, my medical team, our women friends, and all who shared in my journey.

At 8:03 we heard, "It's a GO!" Five minutes later I received a call from Vicki, my primary nurse practitioner. "Linda, I can't be with you. I am at home packing for a trip to Hawaii with my husband." How thoughtful of her to make that call! She reassured me that my team had worked hard to be ready for my surgery, studying what had happened during and after my 2004 bypass surgery. Vicki insisted they were ready for any scenario that might arise.

Although I knew I was in good hands with Kristi, NP, of course I looked forward to seeing Vicki after her vacation. Vicki ended the call with a funny remark. She said Dr. Adamson, my surgeon, had said to her, "If Linda can't wear her purple socks in the operating room, I will wear them."

Kristin learned the latest news when she called at 8:30. Then came the neck-to-knee shaving and scrubbing. By 9:10, Diane and I were still telling stories and being silly.

Finally, at 10:00 I was wheeled to the OR area, wearing my purple socks. Diane was allowed to go with me to the third floor, the OR hallway … for more waiting. This wait gave us a few serious and private moments.

> Diane's Words
>
> We did a short meditation together … Linda was able to say a last "goodbye" to her tired and weary heart … thanking it for serving her well … for so many precious years … and, especially, for seeing her through her most

> *critical times ... until this moment ... as a most*
> *precious gift ... from the heavens ... and from a*
> *kind and gentle soul, one she has yet to learn*
> *about ... has come to support her with a new life*
> *energy ....*
>
> *Linda said she feels her life has already been*
> *very full and so very blessed ... and with grati-*
> *tude and great hope ... she surrenders ... to*
> *whatever the outcome of her heart transplant ...*
> *we asked that all those who care for her...and*
> *make decisions for her ... continue to be di-*
> *vinely guided ... as she trusts in the wisdom and*
> *skill of her surgical team. It was an unforget-*
> *table moment, filled with absolute peace.*

Dr. Adamson arrived. He was kind and reassuring about the new heart. "It's just wonderful, and it is at a nearby hospital. Two of my team members are on their way to examine it. They will bring it to this OR if all is well." He confirmed that he had told Vicki he would wear my purple socks if I wasn't allowed to wear them.

I seriously doubted that he would wear them, but I was amused that he mentioned my special socks. Aren't surgeons supposed to be the serious tunnel-vision, thinking-not-feeling members of the medical team?

Our next visitor was the anesthesiologist, Dr. Corey. He began with, "Hi, I'm Dr. Corey, but you can call me Paul."

"Well, my ex-husband's name is Paul," I said. "I think I will call you Dr. Corey."

"That's fine with me." He was another gentle, kind person. He explained his role on my transplant team and helped me understand what I was likely to experience with the anesthesia.

Can you believe this? I was about to head into the OR to receive a heart transplant. The atmosphere was light and a bit silly. There must have been a note at the top of my chart saying, This patient thrives on humor.

At 10:20 I finally went into the OR, and Diane went to the main lobby to rest and wait for further information.

Diane said she looked up at 10:55, when she realized that Dr. Adamson was approaching in his green scrubs. He quickly told her that everything was fine ... but ... they had decided to wait until morning to do the surgery. The reason had to do with the donor's blood-sodium level being quite high. He said that wouldn't compromise the heart surgery, but that the donor's other organs would benefit and be ready for transplantation to other people if the sodium level was lowered before the surgery.

I felt better hearing that the heart that was potentially mine would also help other people receive donated organs. Surgery was scheduled for 6:00 the next morning. Diane called Kristin. I hoped Kristin and Diane could get some sleep now that they understood the reason for the delay. A corner of the lobby with a padded bench and two loveseats became Diane's bedroom. Yes, she did sleep.

Diane was gently awakened on Sunday (April Fools' Day!) by Andrea, an ICU nurse, at 7:05 in the morning. She gave Diane the good news that the sodium level had improved, but they were still in a holding pattern. The new start time was 10:00am. She added that I had been restless, slept little, and developed an itchy case of hives. Andrea said she had massaged my feet for two hours straight, trying to help me relax.

Of course, Diane called Kristin with the update of more delay.

At 8:00 Diane was taken to the seventh floor "family room." It had a bathroom with a shower, linens, a TV, a chair, and a small foldout bed with a one-inch-thick pad. The lobby "bed" was more comfortable, Diane thought, but she appreciated the quiet, private, dark room.

After Diane ate a light breakfast while I was still pre-op, she found my bed in the third-floor unit, separated from the other patients by just a curtain. She took over the foot and leg massaging. She wrote in her notes that exhaustion was the mood; no more talking. Diane's nursing background proved to be an asset for me. She knew to request glycerin mouth swabs to help with my dry and thirsty state, and a few ice chips to calm my hunger pangs.

Dr. Adamson came in with a different anesthesiologist at 10:15 for a second round of pre-op talks. At 10:40 we were off to surgery. This time, it was for real! Diane said I was still smiling. Soon I was laughing, for the current anesthesiologist said, "Dr. Corey was with you last night, right?"

"Yes," I replied.

"I knew it because Dr. Corey uses so much tape."

Diane was warned that the call to announce that surgery had started would not come for at least an hour. She went to her car to charge her cell phone.

Diane's Words

*One thing for certain, throughout my involve-
ment here, everyone ... the transplant team, the
ICU nurses, nursing and hospital staff ... have
all been respectful and so considerate of me as
Linda's family representative. They've guided,
made allowances, informed, and communicat-
ed with me every step of the way ... forward steps,
back steps, and a side step or two! ... easing the
journey for all. The outcome at every benchmark
has been medically favorable for Linda, so
my job of reporting to family was eased ... and
actually a joy!*

It was 12:25pm when the first news came that the surgery was progressing well. The two team members had just left to pick up and transport
the new heart. Again, Diane was told that it was at a nearby hospital. She
had begun to believe that it was here! "I had a strong feeling about that,"
she told me later.

Diane had some lunch and a two-hour nap on the thin mattress,
thanks to the silence and darkness in the private room.

The best news came when Diane's cell phone awakened her at 3:30 in
the afternoon. Great news! The message from Dr. Adamson was that the
heart was in place. She learned that I had been removed from the heart/
lung machine that had oxygenated and circulated my blood during the
transplant procedure. The new heart was beating on its own! So far, everything looked excellent: vital signs, organ function, blood gasses/chemistry,
and no signs of bleeding.

I got a kick out of Diane's clever use of ((((Heart))) design to designate
the new heart.

Diane's Words on Sunday, April 1, 2007

*4:35 pm, Sunday, Main Lobby - Dr. Adamson
is broadly smiling as he approaches, still in
green scrubs ... everything looks just great! ... the
(((Heart))) is excellent, the medicines used to
avoid past problems have worked out beautifully. He plopped down on a chair and appeared
quite tired, but still very pleased ... and his
words were reassuring.*

> Dr. Adamson said, "How she (Linda) was holding on is just amazing with the condition she had ... her heart was absolutely shot!! I don't know how she was doing it. It was just shot. It's a good thing we went in and the heart became available now ... (he held his hands out to show me how large her sick heart was!). What a wonderful woman she is, and has been throughout this whole ordeal ... she handled it in such an amazing way last night."

Diane called Kristin right away to give her the glowing report. Kristin sounded relieved and happy. She said she and Craig were working on the plans for who would visit and when. Kristin said she would send out a group email message with the happy announcement. She was pleased to learn that she was welcome to call the ICU anytime, day or night.

It was 8:40 that evening when Diane was invited to do the ten-minute scrub for the reverse isolation visit (a method of keeping germs away from the patient) with paper gown, mask, and gloves.

> *Diane's Words*
>
> Linda is all wired up ... leads, tubes, lights, screen, alarm, scopes everywhere ... marking, measuring, computing, IV pushes of who knows what! Lab draws ... and they keep saying "It's fine, you're not in the way ... you can stay as long as you like, sit, stand, whatever" ... Linda is deeply under and out! ... while her new heart is ticking along, running the show. I am amazed, curious, reflective, and nostalgic all at the same time ... my own deja vu, as a nurse, throughout this whole experience ... and I'm honored to be witness to this modern present ... at the same time ... life is so precious, so fragile.

Diane stopped by the hospital for a short visit at 8:00 Monday evening, April 2nd. Just before she went home, she stopped to see me in the ICU. I was awake and off the ventilator, but I still had a tube in my mouth and couldn't talk. In her call to Kristin, Diane said, "Your mother showed big enthusiasm and indicated that she knew she had her new heart." She added, "The nurse said her lung test showed she needed more time on the ventilator."

Thus I was put back "under." I had an interesting experience during this second "down under" time. My memory of that period is very clear. On the other hand, I have no memory of the short time Diane was with me.

This is my vivid recollection of what happened next. I'm ninety-nine-point-nine percent sure it was not a dream, but I wish it had been. The room was dark. I became aware that a male nurse was fiddling with some tape on my left arm. Whatever he was trying to do, he clearly was not succeeding. I was irritated that he seemed to be confused and frustrated, but I stopped worrying about that when I realized the glycerin moisturizing stick was deep in my throat. I couldn't bring my hand to my mouth to pull out the stick.

My anxiety grew as I tried to indicate that I wanted the nurse to get that stick out of my mouth. He looked right at me when I mouthed, "Get help!" but he did not leave the room. I think he may have said, hours later, "I can't take the tube out yet." If I did hear him say that, I didn't understand what he meant. I just wanted the stick out of my mouth. I was terribly agitated, thinking that this inept nurse was keeping me from my surgery.

I don't know how long this went on. He seemed to be backing further and further away from me. Men! They never ask for help. Why wouldn't he just go get someone who knew what to do?! He just let me suffer. I was sure that whatever he was or was not doing was delaying my heart transplant surgery. The next thing I knew, I was gesturing a naughty phrase in sign language that involved my long, straight middle finger. I was beyond frustration. Poor Diane was still waiting in the lobby. Had it been three days already?

I had to help that nurse gain some compassion. He did seem to understand my gesture to come closer. Cautiously, he moved toward me. I grabbed his hand and brought it to my chest. I wanted him to feel my old heart, to feel that I was a real person who was very sick and needed help. A bond was formed. I think he even gave me a hug.

I remember hearing him say he had to leave. He smiled and said he would be my night nurse again. I think I mustered a smile, but my inner voice muttered a sarcastic "Great."

Again, I don't know how much time passed before I was aware of being in a room filled with daylight. Someone was talking to me about pulling the tube out of my throat. As soon as the tube was out, I burst into a tirade about that inept nurse who wouldn't help me. I think I even got in my concern that Diane had been waiting too long in the lobby before the nurse in the room cut me off, saying, "Calm down, calm down. You have a new heart!"

"What?"

"Calm down! You have a new heart!"

That was on Tuesday, April 3rd. I'm not sure what happened next. Once I fully understood what the nurse was saying, I was filled with embarrassment and guilt. I finally realized I'd not had a moisturizing stick caught in my throat. It was a ventilator tube that was helping me breathe. Maybe my long-suffering nurse had been securing the tape that held various IVs in place. No one has ever filled me in on any details as to what I was doing when I was so agitated. I now picture myself thrashing around wildly.

When I began to sort out what had happened, I thought of the beautiful words I knew other transplant patients had said when they became aware they had survived the transplant surgery: "I'm alive!" "Thank God, I made it!" and "I will be able to watch my child grow up now!" I, however, will always have the memory of my not-so-appreciative words, "My nurse was inept, and he wouldn't get help." I was filled with guilt until the staff helped me see the humor in what had happened.

I don't know whether putting me under had involved morphine. I've heard that patients can become quite strong and wild under the influence of morphine. Drugs can be helpful, but the side effects are something else.

Before the next night shift, I told my day nurse to prepare Jason, the "inept nurse," for the huge "I'm sorry and thank you for not putting me in a straightjacket" hug I wanted to give him when he arrived. "Tell Jason I had no idea I already had my new heart," I pleaded. I also sincerely hoped Jason hadn't been able to "read" my naughty hand sign. I have arthritis in my hands, so there's a pretty good chance I'd been unable to curl the necessary fingers while leaving the middle finger straight. Please, arthritis, let that be the time you worked to my advantage by not letting me make that naughty sign.

Not long after they took the breathing tube out of my mouth, my room phone rang. The nurse stepped in and said, "It's your daughter. Pick up the phone." Kristin had called early that morning and learned that I was "still under."

"Kristin?" ... pause ... "Kristin?"

"Is that you, Mommy?"

She was blown away when I started right in, talking at my usual rapid rate of speech. "Yes. I'm sitting in a chair, and I can be here for an hour and a half."

We chatted for at least thirty minutes. I told her the upsetting story about my nasty behavior toward my nurse when I hadn't known I already had my new heart. We laughed, and then I was able to express my sincere understanding and appreciation for the amazing gift I had received. Kristin wrote in her email to the group that "the drugs may have made her act like a lunatic, but Mom sounded normal and excited when I talked with her."

Meanwhile, the nurse had notified Diane that the tube was out and that I was alert and talking.

"Please tell her I'm on my way," Diane replied.

> *Diane's Words*
>
> *Now I'm assuming Linda probably has a very sore throat from the endo tube ... wouldn't it be affirming if I could call Kristin ... let her know I actually witnessed her mom, awake and functioning with her new (((Heart)))?*
>
> *2:30pm, Tuesday, less than 36 hours post-op, I arrive on the scene ... I buzz on the visitor's phone ... walk into the unit ... I look into her glass-enclosed ICU cubicle ... and see Linda sitting straight up in bed! She's grinning like crazy ... and starts waving a piece of broccoli at me, hurrying me to come in! Ohmygosh ... she's eating broccoli??*
>
> *For the "reverse isolation" ICU room today, I only need to do a three-minute hand/arm scrub, put on the gown and mask, and "glove-up" in those bright purple disposables—I'm a bit teary and am TOTALLY in awe over this whole amazing thing! I'm excited to see Linda so bright and alert ....*
>
> *Her first words to me as I walk in? ... "Ask the nurse if you can bring in my camera ... it's over there (she points outside the cubicle door to a*

> bag I recognize, containing all of her personal
> items) ... so, "dutifully," I ask the question ... the
> nurse hesitates ... and then says, "Okay, but only
> you should handle it (the camera), and stay by
> the door ... don't go all the way in ... .

Diane went on to write about the movie scene with me as the director, telling her what to film.

> "Did you get all the wires and tubes, the breath-
> ing machine, the photo poster? I'll toast for the
> camera ... Look! Here comes Dr. Adamson."
>
> Dr. A. started hamming it up and playing right
> along. It's real. Linda's B-A-C-K!

Diane's notes, on lavender paper in the shiny red folder, end with:

> I am deeply honored to have been a trusted
> witness for Linda and her family at this spirit-
> filled juncture on her life path. I will remember
> it always ... I hope we laugh and tell stories for
> a long time to come.

I'm sorry to have to write that Diane was unable to meet Craig or Kristin during their visits. Diane was horrified to realize that she was coming down with a cold. She knew she couldn't come near me with her germs. (Dr. Adamson had the same problem. During one of his visits, he said he could not come into my room because he had a cold.)

My family and I couldn't thank Diane enough for being with me during that wondrous time in our lives!

24

Can You Sashay?

During a phone call from Craig's family in Singapore, five-year-old Tori asked me, "Grandma, how do you like your new heart? Can you jump?" What a great question!

I talked by phone with Ron and Vicki, and they sent out an email with the latest news, namely, that there had been just a few little glitches. At one point my throat had locked up, so I was only able to eat soft foods for a while. The only pain I experienced was sharp, but in short spurts. It was in the upper left side of my chest, where the pacemaker/defibrillator unit had been prior to the transplant surgery. I was told that my body didn't know how to handle the space that had suddenly appeared. All was fine after a day or two with the aid of a light painkiller.

On April 9th, Tony, my physical therapist (who told me that PT stands for Pain and Torture), took me outside my ICU room. A small audience watched me take some cautious steps. Then a male nurse asked me if I could sashay.

"Hmmm?"

"Can you sashay?" he repeated. I proceeded to sway my hips a bit as I walked and he began to sing, "A pretty girl is like a melody." I burst into a laugh. He was singing the song played during the *Miss America Pageants,* I think.

What can I tell you? I loved this place!

After my surgery, I heard no mention of any problem with Heparin. I had been warned that there would be a point during the surgery when it would be used, just as it had been during my bypass surgery in 2004.

Later, looking over my heart transplant hospital records, I saw that Heparin-induced thrombocytopenia had been detected on April 9th. Several tests before that date had shown no detection. After that date, Heparin was not mentioned. As far as I know, it did not rear its ugly head.

There was only one other reference to it: in my Discharge Summary was the statement, "Due to her Heparin allergy, no Lovenox[1] will be provided as part of her therapy."

* * *

A bit later, I was transferred to 7 North, where I had been prepped for my surgery. The move was a good sign that I was progressing well. The fun really began when I settled in. On April 10th, I had phone calls from Omana, Dr. Heywood's nurse practitioner, and from friends and family members. I learned that Vicki, my NP who had gone to Hawaii instead of catering to me, was back home. I couldn't wait to see her.

April 11th was special because that was the day I had my first of many biopsies. Yea! There were no signs of rejection. I enjoyed calls from Kristin and my sister, Marilyn. Tony had me walking down the long hall, turning my head from side to side and reading signs on the walls. We were both pleased that I had no trouble climbing ten stairs, foot over foot, barely holding on to the bannister. I liked walking with my good-looking PT. He dismissed me way too soon.

On Tuesday, the 12th, I looked up and laughed when a happy-face balloon and a big, fuzzy, cuddly teddy bear were delivered. Who would send a hospitalized sixty-six-year-old lady a teddy bear? Dr. Heywood, of course! Years later, I asked him whose idea it had been to give me a teddy bear. He said it was a joint decision with Omana and Brenda, his secretary. "You weren't allowed to have flowers, so ... ." (Live flowers and plants could carry insects and bacteria that might harm very ill or immune-suppressed patients.)

I was happy to hear that JoAnn would come to see me on the 13th. I was so excited to see her that I put on my mask and walked to the elevator, carrying my big teddy bear. I coaxed her to videotape me climbing the stairs. That made her nervous. I can still hear her saying, "Don't you scare me!"

Later that day I had a lesson in checking my blood-sugar level, because one of my medicines could lead to a diabetic-like condition. Samantha, my nurse, had to hold my shaking hand while I tried to prick myself. Once I returned home, I would be testing my blood-sugar level several times a day. It wouldn't take me long to be comfortable with the process.

---

[1] Lovenox (enoxaparin) is an anticoagulant that helps prevent the formation of blood clots. It should not be used if the patient is allergic to Heparin.

I also had the "fun" of learning how to give myself a shot in a flabby area of my tummy. No problem finding a flabby spot. Giving the shot took a bit of courage. The things I said I'd never do! We look at the trials other people have faced and think, "I couldn't do that." Even though I had thought of myself as a bit of a wimp, I did rise to the occasion. All I had to do was remember what everyone had done to get me through this medical adventure. I had to hold up my end of the bargain. My WomenHeart red scarf, my purple socks, and my big teddy bear were always on or near me, inspiring courage.

On April 14th, Nurse Marguerita washed my hair and spiffied up my room in anticipation of a visit from Ron, Vicki, and Jason. They had to wear masks during our long visit. We walked in the hall, and Ron took photos to share with my email group. He gave them a glowing eyewitness report on me and my recovery.

Craig arrived from Singapore late that night. The next day, he and I listened as Vicki, NP, explained about setting out my pills. There were twenty-six different pills in a variety of sizes and colors, and I had to take more than one a day of some of them. Carefully, I put the pills in my huge, bright-blue-edged seven-day pill box—forty-four per day, shining like tiny Easter eggs in their proper time slots. What an interesting and time-consuming project! There were pills to reduce the reaction of my immune system so my body wouldn't reject my new heart. Each pill played a role in keeping me healthy or in minimizing the side effects of my many medications.

Organizing my meds helped me realize how grateful I was for the research done at Stanford University and other centers around the world. I'm grateful for the scientists who developed techniques for detecting organ rejection, discovered new medicines, and learned how the medications interact with each other. They persevered in the studies that made organ transplantation safer and allowed transplant patients to live longer, healthier lives.

＊ ＊ ＊

Marilyn A. sent me a funny email. She said my tales of hospital life reminded her of the "Queen for a Day" TV show. The theme of the show had involved crowning a deserving Miss or Mrs. Jane Q. Public. Amid much fanfare, "the Queen" was showered with exciting presents. Servants glamorized her for one day, brought her fancy meals, and did her daily chores. My depiction of my extended stay sounded to Marilyn like one big party, with lots of good-looking males on my medical team meeting my every need!

One quiet evening, I requested to go to the ICU to give personal thank-yous and take photos. My nurse agreed to push me there in a wheelchair.

I was especially happy to see and hug Jason, "my inept nurse," as well as the nurse who had sung to me as I sashayed in the ICU. We ended my outing by lingering at the nurses' station near my room. Amid lots of light talking, I heard, "You're enjoying this, aren't you?" With a huge smile and a laugh, I said, "Yes!" I had touching interactions with my nurses. Even the male nurses proudly showed me photos of their children.

On April 17th, Craig came to listen to the exit lessons.

I had one more heart biopsy. The biopsies were performed under local anesthesia and took about twenty minutes. Using a catheter that went in through my neck, the doctor was able to snatch tiny pieces of my heart. Those pieces were sent to the lab to check for signs of rejection.

I was fortunate that my biopsies showed no signs of rejection. I was back in my home by 4:30 on Tuesday afternoon, April 17th, 2007.

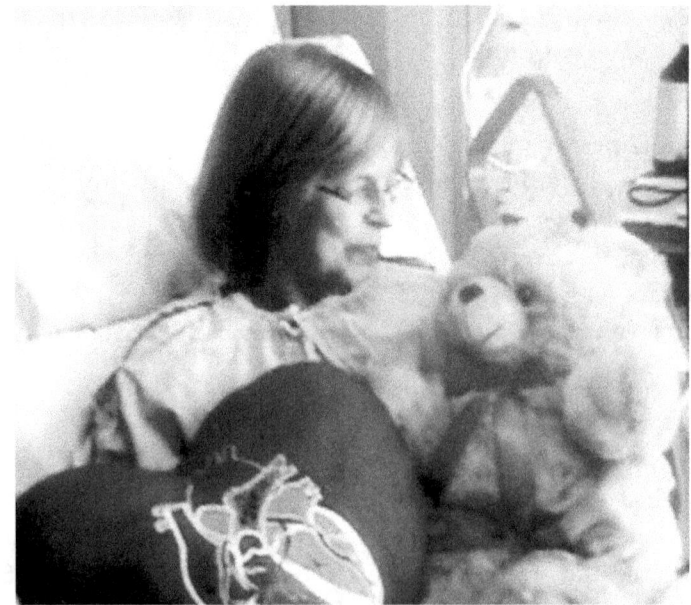

Grateful for healthy new heart, heart pillow, big teddy bear

25

Bait and Switch

"Bait and switch" is the phrase that comes to mind for my transition from hospital to home. During my last days at the hospital I was walking down the hall alone, talking with everyone and grinning from ear to ear. I was euphoric about having a new heart and a chance to be a new and better person. I felt strong. Invincible.

As soon as Craig parked the car, I started to bolt up the stairs to visit my next-door neighbors. Whoa! I quickly slowed my gait and began to pull myself up the long flight of steps, hand over hand on the railing, to reach the landing. A bit of huffing and puffing snuck in on me as well. Uh oh. Walking up a real flight of steps had left me a bit wobbly. I got it—I had some recovering to do. My visit with Peggy and Joe was worth the effort that accompanied this awakening to my new reality.

April 18th was my first full day at home. The visiting nurse arrived early to guide me through the post-transplant home routines and "rules." She was pleasant until she learned that my daughter would arrive the next day with her two young children.

"Young children will be staying here?!" She softened her tone, but impressed upon Craig and me the seriousness of germ vulnerability for immunosuppressed patients. Bottles of hand sanitizer were placed in every room of my home and in my car. The nurse had done a good job of making it clear that germs were forbidden to come near me!

✳ ✳ ✳

Craig left for the airport the next night. I became concerned around nine o'clock when Kristin and her children still hadn't arrived. A few minutes later, I heard the car pull up. Then the front door opened. In came Aengus. He gave me a quick wave and headed to the bathroom, calling out, "Hi, Grandma! I'm going to wash my hands to help keep your new heart healthy." Craig brought in our sleeping Petra and took her to the waiting bed.

With a huge smile announcing the arrival of her dragging body, in came a tired but enthusiastic Kristin. She squealed her traditional high-pitched "Mommy!" Beyond informing me they had stopped for dinner, her need for sleep took precedence over any desire she might have had to chat.

I awoke the next morning to the hushed sounds of children talking and laughing. I thought of the nurse's plea for caution, but I knew my "health level" had shot up to a new high. Two of my grandchildren were on the other side of the wall. In two months Grace and Tori would be back from Singapore. I would have to balance being near my grandchildren with following every health rule.

Kristin and the children stayed for three weeks. They had many adventures, with and without me. We were in constant contact, thanks to our cell phones.

Laughter Yoga with Gaga and Khevin at South Ponto Beach was my first choice for social activity. We stayed down at beach level, instead of climbing the stairs to the bluff. The traditional "Ho ho ha-ha-ha" chant with rhythmic claps got us started. Kristin jumped right in. Soon we were giggling and then belly-laughing.

The young ones gave us curious looks and then bent down to play in the sand, ignoring the silly adults. When we got home, however, Aengus began doing several of the laughter "exercises" at the top of his lungs as he hopped up and down my indoor stairs. We joined in on his delayed reaction, and he kept us laughing often during the next few days.

I had an interesting situation with Aengus, who was almost four years old. We had been to a park. Petra was asleep when we arrived at home. Kristin left the car to go in and take a shower, and Aengus and I talked in the car while Petra slept. Out of the blue my grandson asked me, "What did they do with your old heart?"

I paused and said, "My heart was very sick. Maybe they threw it away." Aengus didn't comment. Then I said, "I really think my heart was taken to a university to be examined by students who want to become doctors." Aengus's daddy taught at a university, so I felt that explanation would make sense to him.

Later, I shared with Vicki, NP, what I had told Aengus. She approved of my answer.

✷ ✷ ✷

Health-wise, we decided my deck was the best location for hosting relatives and friends who came for short visits.

I was delighted by a visit from one of my ICU nurses. As I sat on the deck waiting for her, down the path she came, holding a pretty flowering plant. I had to laugh. She made a funny face and sputtered, "Oh no, you can't be near plants. I, of all people, should have known that. I know you— you're going to tell everyone, aren't you?!"

I had a long visit with Kim, from Healing Hearts, and Kathy from WomenHeart. The longer I rattled off my favorite funny heart adventure stories, the bigger their eyes grew. We all realized they'd met me during my congestive heart failure stage. Although I'd been outgoing and enthusiastic then, I guess I looked a whole lot healthier during this visit. One of them said I looked twenty years younger than when she'd last seen me.

A few days before Kristin's family left we went to the airport to pick up my sister, Marilyn, who would be taking over as my chief caretaker for the next three weeks. Our next trip to the airport was to meet Brian. What a delight it was to see the joyful family reunion! Petra put on a big show of love for her daddy.

During Marilyn's stint with me, we went to a wedding, a Women-Heart meeting, Sarito's laughing meditation, and medical appointments.

✳ ✳ ✳

Do you remember that I had asked people to guess what day they thought I would get my new heart? Well, one person guessed the correct date! When I'd asked my sister whether she would like to make a guess, she paused and then chose April 1st.

"Really?" I wondered why she'd chosen that date. She might have been thinking of our mother's birthday, which was early in April, but not on the 1st. Not on April Fools' Day.

Marilyn won! I treated her to a massage by my friend and massage therapist, Cindy. She and I had shared a lot of stories, before and after my many massages.

✳ ✳ ✳

During my first outings, I wore a medical facemask. I tried not to feel self-conscious as I went about my errands. I got into many enjoyable conversations with people who asked me about it.

When I was shopping for new clothes, a salesclerk came over to me. I told her about my recent heart transplant surgery. She walked away, and I kept looking at the merchandise.

As I was paying for the item I'd chosen, the clerk handed me a pretty gift-wrapped box. She said the staff wanted me to have a token of their best wishes for my full recovery. I opened the box and saw a beautiful gray-green candle "to light in honor of your new life." What a lovely gesture! I think of the friendly clerks whenever I wear the colorful floral print jacket I purchased that day.

Another day, unexpectedly, I began to cry softly after I'd parked my car and was heading to a bookstore. It was the first of several times I would be suddenly struck by the reality that I was alive and breathing easily with the help of someone else's heart. I could talk and even laugh about it, but I had a hard time, in private, accepting the reality of what had happened between my donor and me.

✶ ✶ ✶

My "bossy" and caring neighbor, Sherin, stopped by often to see whether I was following my doctor's orders. He was right when he accused me of not being serious about resting. I was high on life. I came up with a workable plan that earned his approval. I gave myself the gift of being on my bed with my head slightly raised for two hours a day. I doubted I would fall asleep, so I needed a reason, a hook, or a genuine treat that would keep me on my bed.

That hook turned out to be watching "Oprah" and "Ellen" on TV every day. In the past, I'd considered these shows guilty pleasures in which I could immerse myself only when I was almost caught up on my To-Do list. Ha! In my twisted mind, I was now treating "Oprah" and "Ellen" as medical tax deductions.

Oprah ... Isn't it interesting that we refer to her by her first name, as if she were a trusted friend? Oprah presented a wide range of entertaining, informational, and inspirational programs, from fun with celebrities to opening our awareness of difficult topics. Wasn't it great that I was encouraged to indulge in daytime TV?

As for Ellen DeGeneres, she provided one of my favorite stories. I was on my bed, being a good girl, when Ellen's show opened with her sitting at an incline on a hospital bed. A little to the side stood a good-looking EMT. Why are all paramedics so darned handsome?

Ellen reminded her viewers that she had hurt her back. I think that happened after her many high-jumps over the coffee table on the set, or after playing with her dog. Whatever. She did not want to stop doing her show, so she carried on while sitting on the bed that day and for a few more days.

Ellen started in on a bit that involved shopping in drug stores, looking for odd or intriguing products. Since she couldn't go to the store herself, she'd sent a staff member to do the purchasing. Laughing, I began noting the items she showed. To the best of my note taking, here are the products, minus most of her hilarious quips that had me in stitches:

1. Icy hot packs for her pain

2. A box of chardonnay wine … for longer-lasting pain relief

3. A picnic cooler large enough to keep the box of wine cold

4. A twelve-inch box with a clear bright-blue-edged lid, seven inches wide and an inch and a half high. Picking it up, she said, "Who would need a pill box *this big* for a one-week supply of pills?"

The box looked familiar to me. I looked over my shoulder and answered, "Yo!" My seven-day supply of forty-four pills a day looked back at me from their neat columns, each one divided into four sections (breakfast, lunch, dinner, bedtime).

5. A big, large-print crossword puzzle book

6. An issue of "Oprah" magazine that included an article on pain relief

7. A romance novel, from which Ellen read a juicy part in her sexiest voice.

Fade to commercial.

✶ ✶ ✶

My 2007 lab reports were good, with minor changes in medicines. Better yet, there were no signs of rejection of my new heart. By the beginning of May, I had developed the Cushingoid moon-face appearance, a typical side effect of taking Prednisone, a steroid.

Once the initial red puffiness softened, people began to comment on how healthy I looked. I had to tell them that this slightly rounder look was my "sick face." I sort of preferred the softer, fluffed-out face, which reminded me of my mother. As my Prednisone doses lessened, my face gradually returned to its normal, thin shape.

✶ ✶ ✶

I became fond of my heart transplant cardiologist, Dr. Jaski, just as Dr. Heywood had said I would. During my first few biopsies, I remember asking Dr. J., "Have you started putting in the wire yet?" I was always surprised when he said he was ready to pull out the wire. He was a smooth operator.

During one session, I remember Dr. Jaski telling me about a medical meeting where he had sat next to Dr. Heywood. "What do you think we talked about most?" he asked me. Then he answered, "You!"

I can't remember when I learned the full truth about Dr. Heywood's background. He and Dr. Jaski had been colleagues and friends for many years. I knew Dr. Heywood had worked at Loma Linda University Hospital and had excellent credentials. Eventually, I learned that *he had been their heart transplant cardiologist.*

I think it was good that I hadn't known of his specialty earlier. I have a high fear threshold and might have worried that a heart transplant was a possibility before Dr. Heywood had a chance to choose the optimum time to gently broach the subject.

The transplant cardiologists and nurse practitioners have their hands full and their brains stretched, as each patient reacts differently, both physically and emotionally, to the medicines and the reality of the gift of life they have received.

On one of my first post-transplant office visits, I entered the waiting room and spoke to other patients before seeing Vicki, NP. The NPs hear all the patients' "what's going on" stories. I'm sure most newbies have long lists of questions, tell lengthy tales of dealing with the side effects of their meds, and unload information about whatever emotional roller coaster they are riding that day.

I was told that Dr. Jaski would be in to see me in a few minutes. Followed by Vicki, he entered with a big smile and a cheery greeting. He reached out to shake my hand. Being extra-serious about the new rules I had to live by, especially the one about not touching germy people or things, I instinctively pulled back my hand. With much surprise, Dr. J. turned his head quickly to look at Vicki and asked, "Can't even I touch her?!"

It took several months to convince Dr. J. that I prefer hugs, anyway!

As I left the examining room, I was introduced to a woman who was celebrating twenty-one years with her transplanted heart. Wow! She looked so healthy!

* * *

Sometime in May, Vicki told me that my new heart had come from a teenaged girl. I was not told the circumstances of her death. I drove home from that appointment with a myriad of conflicting thoughts. Filled with grief about the end of a young girl's life, I kept thinking of her family, especially her mother. I ached for her, and admired her for being able and willing to give the lifesaving gift of organ donation at such a difficult time in her own life.

I couldn't help but feel a heavy cloud hanging over my rainbow of gratitude. Pangs of guilt hit me, and I shed many tears during my drive home. Of course, I realized that my medical need was not in any way responsible for her death. Accepting that truth, however, did not lessen the sadness lurking behind my survival. My drive home seemed to take forever.

I asked Vicki when I would be able to write a thank-you letter to my donor's family. She told me to wait a few months.

I told Vicki a story about Diane, my "family" liaison at the time of my surgery. Diane had told me that just before my surgery, she'd had a strong feeling my donor and the family were "right here" in this hospital. Vicki said, "Well, since your donor was a teenager, she was at Rady Children's Hospital, just an overpass walkway from the OR where you were being prepared for your procedure." Diane's intuition had been right.

* * *

By mid-May I was ready to start cardiac rehab. It felt good to get on a treadmill again. I often exercised with a patient who had received his new heart just ten days after I got mine. In the mirror we could see our funny matching moon faces.

On May 29th, after a biopsy appointment, I stopped at Scripps Green Hospital to visit Dr. Heywood and others on my medical team. I was beyond happy, telling them, "Thank you for keeping me alive until I received the gift of renewed health and life!"

Dr. Heywood countered with, "She has the Gratitude Attitude!"

* * *

I returned to taking long walks in my neighborhood, sometimes twice a day. I was pleased one day in June when I succeeded at going up a long, steep grade. But new challenges appeared as well. My weight and glucose levels were going up. The pain from bloating was back. Hadn't I had enough of that before the transplant? Honest, I was following the healthy-eating and exercising tips from the cardiac rehabilitation center.

As the strong new medicines accumulated in my body, I developed a string of typical side effects: weak leg muscles, shaky fingers and hands, a scary (but quickly resolved) dehydration episode, light-headedness, along with feeling too hyper to want to rest during the day and then not being able to relax enough to sleep at night.

* * *

My spirits were high enough that I decided, at the last minute, to attend my forty-fifth college reunion with Occidental College classmates. Dr. Jaski gave his approval for the two-hour drive and a few sips of champagne during the Class of '62 toast!

Still in high spirits during my drive home, I stopped to do a few errands. I had a lively talk with a teddy-bear kind of fellow in Trader Joe's who was helping children find treasures the staff had hidden around the store. As I was checking out, Erik headed toward me with a bouquet of fresh flowers in colors that matched the multicolored printed flowers on my jacket. It was another of the unexpected perks on this medical adventure of mine, a gift from him and the store's staff.

After a visit to a party store, I called JoAnn to tell her about my reunion. I ended with the story about the flowers.

"Um, Linda, you are not supposed to be handling fresh flowers."

"Yikes!" I shouted. "I'd better keep them in the paper wrapping. I'll put the whole bouquet in a big vase and set it on my patio!"

Either the flowers were not full of bad bacteria or I was one strong patient, because here I am, sitting at my computer typing. I had no setbacks from all the lovely plants and flowers that dared come near me.

* * *

So … why had I stopped at the store? I was getting party items for the "I'm Okay" Party suggested by Jim, my friend and financial advisor. My son had said my birthday would be a good day for it. Saturday, July 7, 2007, would be the perfect day to let friends know I had survived heart transplant surgery and was flying high with gratitude!

I struggled at the computer to compose a letter of thanks to my medical teams at the two hospitals. I coupled the thank-you with an invitation to my "I'm Okay" Party for everyone who had supported me physically or emotionally with upbeat comments, laughter opportunities, transportation, home tasks, or errands.

Personally delivering my appreciation letter to my doctors presented one especially meaningful interchange. Yes, I had been unnerved by Dr. Hassidim, hematologist, during my first appointment. But I wanted him to know I was thankful for his thorough research and concern for my health, especially in light of my prior complications during surgery.

He surprised me by saying, "I'm happy that the other doctors did not agree with me about disqualifying you for transplantation."

"Me too," I quickly agreed. I gave him a strong hug.

I had planned to keep a promise to my son that I would not go overboard with my party preparations. That promise was shattered when I got carried away with shopping and thinking of ways to help my guests interact with each other as they looked over the souvenirs I planned to display on the tables.

My scrapbook, titled "My New Heart Adventure," was my most successful project. It included photos taken in both hospitals, emails to and from my supporters, the newspaper article about the 2004 Kentucky Derby, the chunk of hair I'd pulled out of my head after my bypass surgery, and samples of hospital menus, placemats, and the like.

By party day, I had caught a cold and had to wear a mask to keep my germs from my guests, instead of the other way around.

As usual, I had not allowed myself enough time to set up. My condo friends took over, moving tables and chairs and arranging the food and my souvenirs. They became hosts and hostesses, right through to putting away the furniture and vacuuming the rug at the end of the party! Vicki, Ron, and Jason looked on in amazement. For over twenty years they had been the ones to bail me out of my sinking pre-party ships!

✳ ✳ ✳

The date July 7, 2007 ... 07/07/07 ... was touted as a universal lucky day, but it was my real sixty-seventh birthday. While others headed to Las Vegas, got married, and participated in a variety of activities they hoped would bring them good luck, I was floored when sixty-one guests joined me on my Day of Gratitude, several having driven for over an hour to get there.

Some highlights:

• I received a call from Dr. Pressman, my GI doctor, explaining that he'd wanted to attend but had prior plans.

(I'd had no idea any of my doctors or hospital staff members would take my invitation seriously. I was almost speechless when I received the call from Dr. Pressman himself.)

• Emails arrived from two other doctors expressing their regrets; one was heading for Spain.

• My visiting nurse came, as well two nurses from a cardiac clinic.

• Kirkos, the artist who drew soulful labyrinths in the sand for us to walk, was surprised to see many people he knew.

• Guests whispered about seeing "Ambulance Driver" on Sherin's nametag. He thought he deserved the title, since he'd driven me to the hospital to get my new heart.

• People stopped to greet me and then circulated around the room. Happy noise!

• Before I stepped up to talk to the whole group, I danced around the room singing "I Feel Pretty" from the musical *West Side Story*. I swished past my friends in my new lavender blouse and flowing, full-length skirt. I was still wearing my fat face (minus the mask) and bloated tummy, but I had never felt so loved or beautiful, inside and out!

• I had written on the invitation that I would share my favorite stories with everyone. I got off to a rocky start when I introduced some Laughter Yoga exercises. Most guests joined in, but some looked a little nervous about laughing just for the feel-good sensation it brings.

• A glance at the walkway turned me into an instant screaming teenager. "OH, OH, OH! He came! He came!" I'm pretty sure my guests thought I was having a seizure. In walked "my beloved," Dr. Heywood, my cardiologist, dressed casually in a short-sleeved shirt and knee-length shorts. No doctor's coat. He gave me a warm hug.

My onlookers had no idea what was happening. I finally told them who he was and related a few tales about him. Then I turned to him and said, "Where is your wife? I want to meet her." He told us he and his wife were attending another party, but he'd slipped away for a short while to see me.

• I was so high on life and Prednisone that I talked even faster then usual. I was told I was funny to watch, even if my audience couldn't understand a word I said. I know they got the gist of my stories because they were laughing and crying at all the appropriate times.

* * *

A couple of weeks before my party, I had surprised myself by deciding to order special license plates for my car. I wanted to shout out to the universe my thank-you for my heart transplant gift.

I played with the seven spaces allotted by the DMV. I finally settled on:

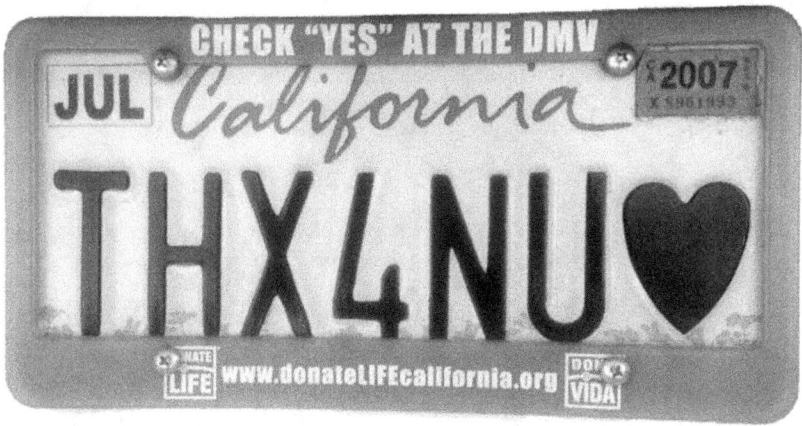

26

For Every Rose, Some Thorns ...

By mid-July, I had discomfort that posed a mystery for several doctors in different specialties. In hindsight, I know that the intense pressure I felt from my neck down to my groin had two sources, rather than just one.

From notes about my ever-changing weight pre- and post-transplant:

During my three years with congestive heart failure ... 119-130 pounds

After my transplant through August of 2007 ... 115-133.5 pounds

Why have I highlighted my weight gain? It was the symptom that alerted us to a mystery that wouldn't be solved until September. During my third month post-transplant, I was keeping up my healthy and enjoyable activities, but I felt miserable. I will only mention Dr. Jaski's name with respect to this issue because he was the one doctor who admitted to being truly perplexed. He did not make me feel like a hypochondriac, as did some of the other doctors.

While the pressure kept increasing throughout my torso, the bloating seemed to be the troublemaker. I was being tossed around among cardiologists, gastroenterologists, urgent care doctors, and my primary care physician.

My morale was tested by doctors' comments and, later, by reading the following entries found in medical notes from several doctors:

"She complains of persistent abdominal bloating, self-medicating with Lasix when her weight goes over 120."

"Has vague abdominal symptoms from meds or IBS ... see a GI doctor."

"You have to understand that the first six months post-surgery are the hardest."

"Weight 128; no appreciable fluid in abdomen; overall she feels great, except the bloating pressure."

On July 19th, I told my new GI doctor about my painful abdominal bloating that built up during the day. I told him I felt miserable at night, that my belly was rigid, my fingers tingly, my hands shaky; I reported numbness in my breasts and a bloated feeling right after eating even a small amount. I told him that Drs. Jaski and Heywood had said I was dehydrated. After looking at scans taken before my transplant, the GI doctor said, "It is just the fluid, so take diuretics!"

I did not like that doctor's manner. I never saw him again.

They did an ultrasound: no problems with internal organs, no calculi, no pockets of water.

Notes from my new primary care physician, July 30th

She feels like she is swollen and bloated, mostly upper abdomen; dull pressure; no diarrhea or constipation, some flatulence; no chest pain; let's try Prevacid or maybe Levbid; then go back to the GI doctor.

During one appointment I heard, "We can find nothing wrong, and it is not for a lack of trying. We *are* trying to help you! You are a recent transplant patient. Your body is not the same. You can't expect to be as strong or have the weight you had years ago. You probably aren't exercising as much."

Meanwhile, my son said I should see a toxicologist or someone who studied the interaction of the medicines a person was taking. He had seen in my notes that whenever my dose of Prednisone, a steroid, went down, my dose of Neoral, an immunosuppressant, went up. Hmm … .

In a letter to a friend on August 8th, I wrote, "I will go to Urgent Care tomorrow. No one thinks it is a heart problem. I've had scans and an ultrasound. The chest pressure came on slowly until last Thursday. I have gained three pounds in three days. Craig thinks it is drug-related, especially with Neoral. My cardiologists want me to see GI doctors.

I had hoped to be admitted to the hospital; I got upset when the Scripps Urgent Care doctor said, "It's just fluid buildup."

He also said my weight might be from my new appetite and being on Prednisone, and that Neoral should not be a problem. I asked why. I think he said that was because it wouldn't get into the system.

In another letter to my friend I wrote,

What can I do? I'm too tired to look for some decent flowing clothes, especially long pants with loose elastic at the waist. I need bigger bras that won't press on my larger and very tender breasts. Poor, Pitiful Me!

But, no fear; I am already laughing about yesterday's Urgent Care visit. The doctor said, "You won't die from bloating!" He couldn't imagine feeling, as I did, like he was about to deliver twins or triplets! I have promised to rest, skip working with my trainer, and take shorter walks.

I promised Craig I would record everything that has to do with my food, drugs, and activities.

My weight was higher than either of my full-term pregnancy weights!

On August 10th, I had an echocardiogram. My EF "score" was 73.534%. Wow!!! That was way above average for a woman my age! My new heart had settled in beautifully.

An August 16th CT scan of my chest and abdomen showed slight constipation but no obstruction.

Meanwhile, I was functioning pretty well. I was attending my evening women's circle meetings and support groups. I had a wonderful visit with Karen, a friend from my teaching days in LaVerne, and another visit with Vicki and Ron. I spent time with my granddaughters, enjoyed a Kundalini Dancing session with Sarito, and gave a thank-you dinner party at our favorite Italian restaurant for my Crazy Condo friends.

* * *

On August 27th my primary care physician said, "Linda, there is nothing more we can do for you!"

Can you imagine how it felt to have my doctors all throwing up their hands, most of them convinced I was exaggerating my symptoms? The pain I was experiencing was the worst I had felt since embarking on this heart journey back in 2004. It was definitely physical pain, augmented by my emotional distress.

At the same time, I did believe my doctors cared and wanted to find a solution. I knew that Dr. Jaski took me seriously when he commented, "I'm sorry we are just tossing you off to each other."

An interesting twist occurred shortly after my August 27th visit to my primary care provider. I was standing near a drugstore pharmacist's window when a book caught my eye. *The Pill Book* was billed as "new and revised 12th edition of the illustrated guide to the most-prescribed drugs in the United States."

Standing in the store aisle, I began my research. On page 333, I found the information about Neoral, the brand name for Cyclosporine, the immunosuppressant I was taking to prevent rejection of transplanted organs. There were six pages of definitions, uses, cautions and warnings, possible side effects, drug interactions, and so on. In what follows, I have italicized the symptoms mentioned there that I was experiencing:

Mild symptoms usually *start after about 2 or 3 months of treatment.*

Under the category of possible side effects:

• Most common: known to be toxic to the kidneys, high blood pressure, *increased hair growth,* and enlargement of the gums

• Less common: tremors, cramps, acne, *tingling in the hands or feet,* headache, confusion, *facial flushing, swollen and painful male breasts, fluid retention and swelling,* ringing or buzzing in the ears, and more.

• Rare: yada, yada, yada.

Wait, back up—*SWOLLEN AND PAINFUL MALE BREASTS???*

After buying the book, I practically ran home. Okay, I drove home. I couldn't get to the phone fast enough.

"I think I have swollen and painful male breasts under my breasts, causing severe pain in my own breasts." It was probably to Kathy, the ever-pleasant heart transplant office receptionist, that I blurted my news. I don't think I spoke to Dr. Jaski that day.

As soon as was possible, I asked Dr. Jaski, "Can I switch from Neoral to Prograf?" (Prograf, the brand name for Tacrolimus, is another immunosuppressant used to prevent organ rejection.) Like a whining young child, I said, "You let Cathleen change to Prograf. Can I?" Cathleen and I had both experienced increased growth of body hair as a side effect of our medicine. The extra-fine blond hair on my face and arms wasn't as noticeable as was Cathleen's dark hair.

Dr. Jaski said he would consider my request. On September 4th, five months after my transplant and three months after the bloating began, Dr. Jaski told me I could stop Neoral and try Prograf.

I took my first Prograf pills on September 10th, morning and evening.

At my next GI doctor appointment, I cancelled the upper-GI scan because I was sure I had found the source of the extreme pressure in my chest.

While I had a slight problem with low blood pressure, I had fewer face flushes and *no* painful pressure in my chest—just eight days after starting Prograf! My "painful and swollen male breasts" were gone, and never came back.

The odd thing is that my "own" breasts stayed larger than they had been pre-transplant. I was finally more in line with the rest of the females in my family. Ha! I got a new heart and a boob job!

I made copies of page 333 of *The Pill Book* and gave them to each of the doctors I'd seen during my medical ordeal. Dr. Jaski gets five stars! He is the *only* doctor who made any comment about the solution I found.

At my next biopsy appointment, Dr. Jaski said, "I have been working with heart transplant patients for over twenty years. I have never heard of a patient who experienced that side effect."

Thank goodness, after years of research, there are a variety of medications for most of our conditions. While one pill does wonders for many patients, there always seem to be a few patients who experience negative reactions. In defense of doctors, I want to say I have always felt that it was part science and part miracle that they can help their patients get relief, become cured, or learn how to cope with an unlimited range of medical possibilities.

I believe strongly in the mind-body connection. The body may be "fixed," but if the mind doesn't agree, the mental and physical pain may continue. On the plus side, there are people who have survived dire situations and conditions when the "facts" indicated that death or no relief was expected.

Here's a story about the other Neoral side effect I had experienced: In the hospital, we were given information about our pills and what could happen when taking them. Increased hair growth was mentioned. I'm not talking about extra hair on your head; I could have used extra hair there. I'm talking about new hair all over the body ... not so pretty.

My extra hair was almost white, like the baby hair I'd grown soon after birth. In bright light, I could see the fuzz appearing on my face and arms. Grace and Tori became fascinated with my soft, furry skin. They liked to stroke my face. I told them about the medicine I took. They didn't seem to be concerned.

As they were about to get in the car to leave my home, I said, "Guess what! I think I am turning into a teddy bear. I'm fuzzy, and I love hugs." They looked at me seriously at first and then one of them said, "Grandma, you're silly!"

27

Where Did They Find Your New Heart?

Soon after Vicki, NP, had told me my new heart had come from a teenage girl, she'd given me a brochure from Life Sharing, the San Diego affiliate of the California organization, Donate Life. In it were guidelines for writing a thank-you letter. As sensitively as possible, I wanted to convey my gratitude for my donor family's gift to me.

I'm not certain when I gave my letter to Vicki to pass on to Life Sharing. A representative would deliver it to my donor's family. On October 16th, as she was prepping me for my biopsy, Vicki said gently, "I have something special for you." From her lab coat pocket she pulled out an envelope and handed it to me.

The letter had been written by my donor's mother. She described her daughter and the rest of the family, and said she would like to meet me. I was deeply moved when I read that I had helped her with her grieving. Learning that some good had come from her loss had a cathartic effect on me. I felt a warm connection had begun.

I wrote back to tell her I would very much like to meet her. The Life Sharing organization would set up a meeting that would include a nurse or other professionals who could provide us emotional support. I suggested that she take her time to decide when she would be ready to meet me.

I realized that meeting my donor's family could be an emotionally charged event for all of us. I wanted them to feel my deep sense of gratitude, but I was concerned about the pain they might suffer.

I'm sad to say that I haven't had the opportunity to meet my donor's family. I have chosen to assume they did not want to relive the tragedy. I visualize my donor being with me as I accept new challenges. I do know her name. I will respect her family's privacy by not telling more about her, since I wasn't able to ask for permission to share specific information.

* * *

The American Heart Association's mid-September San Diego Heart Walk was extra special for me in 2007. It was my third time walking, but my first time walking with another person's heart. In spite of all the light-hearted moments I've experienced and written about, I have always remained mindful of the source of my physical and emotional well-being.

For the first time, my son's family was able to be with me. We walked the Survivors' (Red Hat) Walk, a short version of the main event. As we crossed the finish line, strolling and laughing with others who had also taken the no-stress route, I was approached by an NBC news photographer. We had a short conversation. After milling around for a while, I saw the photographer coming toward me again. He asked whether I would like to be interviewed on live television. Me? Talk? Sure. My son laughed and warned the man, "She does like to talk!"

With my family looking on, I asked the reporter whether I could mention that I'd done the Heart Walk with my doctor last year, and that two months later I'd been put on the Heart Transplant Waiting List. It was a short interview, but I managed to express gratitude for my medical teams from two hospitals and for my donor's family, as well as tell about walking with my doctor.

Later in the day, I learned that my friend Marilyn A. had seen the interview. She knew me well, knew how fast I talked when I was nervous. Her rave review meant a lot to me. She insisted I'd spoken slowly and clearly enough and had gotten all my points across. I was on TV, and I didn't make a fool of myself!

✶ ✶ ✶

About a week later, I attended an evening Heart Transplant Support Group meeting. Walking from my car to the meeting room, I put on my germ-barring mask. We didn't have to wear our masks in the meeting room. There were only four transplant survivors, someone's father, another person's wife, our new leader (a social worker), and a nurse-practitioner trainee. This time there were no pre-transplant patients.

The discussion was heavier than usual. It wasn't a gripe session, but it was a safe place for attendees to do deeper sharing concerning the side effects of the medicines and the financial strain of the cost of the medicines and other expenses, such as the gas to get to our many appointments. We shared more about the emotional roller coaster ride of gratitude for our lifesaving gift and the negative thoughts about the challenges we still faced.

Toward the end of the meeting, I developed a strong headache. I needed to take something for my pain before driving home. I put my mask back on as I left the meeting. I didn't have any pain-relieving drug; the hospital gift shop was closed, and I couldn't get anything from the ER.

I headed for my car, got in, and started to cry. I was overloaded with our emotional sharing. It was drizzling during my drive home via three freeways. My head was splitting, tears ran down my face, and my vision blurred because it was dark and my glasses were fogging up. Traffic was moving fast. Driving in the light rain was difficult during the freeway transitions. I was scared about my driving conditions, and concerned about the other patients.

My forty-five-minute drive was almost over. I made my exit to the right, and then moved quickly to the left lane for the upcoming turn. Making my left turn onto the quiet street, I realized I was still wearing my hospital mask. No wonder my glasses had been fogging up! Every time I exhaled, the mask would push my warm breath straight up into my eyes and glasses.

I began to laugh and cry at the same time. I did not want to go to my empty house. I needed to talk to someone, anyone. I longed to be with a friend. I drove slowly past the homes of two friends. No lights on. Though I didn't want to disturb JoAnn, who got up and out early in the morning, I hoped her light was still on. I always felt comfortable talking with her.

Driving past JoAnn's condo, I saw a light in her kitchen. I parked my car in my garage and walked up the stairs to her front door. She took one look at me and hurried to open the door. What would I have done without JoAnn? She was so patient. She let me tell about the meeting and my emotional reaction.

"Why do I have it so easy?" I blubbered. I started to say, "When I think of how lucky I am ..." and then I broke into a nervous laugh. "On top of all that," I rattled on, "I drove all the way home with my mask on! I was having such a hard time seeing through the drizzle, you know. I kept wiping the windshield with my hand, but then—I was almost all the way home before I realized I was still wearing the stupid mask. Can you believe it? I jerked it off—and all of a sudden, I could see!"

JoAnn definitely got an earful. JoAnn, JoAnn, JoAnn. I can't thank her enough for being in my life when I needed her!

* * *

In October, my cousin Ed was in San Diego for a medical convention. We spent two days together, talking nonstop while enjoying tourist activities. Our families had gotten together once a year when we were children, and as adults we'd kept in touch across the miles in spite of the demands of our respective occupations and family commitments.

We were both rapid talkers with a wide range of interests and conversation topics. He was a doctor, a practicing and teaching radiologist with many questions about my transplant experience. I delighted in relating my medical tale. We share a similar sense of humor, so he could appreciate my offbeat "take" on even the most serious situations. I loved having such an attentive audience for my memories. After our two days together we began calling more frequently. He was the first person to insist repeatedly that I write down my stories.

∗ ∗ ∗

By November, my energy level made it easy to handle volunteering for holiday projects with several organizations. Early in December I flew to Idaho to be with my daughter's family. We had snow the whole time I was there. The view from the living room window out over snow-topped homes and leafless trees reminded me of scenes I'd seen featured on elegant Christmas cards.

I joined in on several parties and holiday activities. Aengus, my intellectually curious grandson, provided my most interesting memory. He had another zinging question for me:

"Grandma, where did they find your new heart?"

Kristin had not been with us when he'd asked me months earlier, "What did they do with your old heart?" and she wasn't with us this time. Especially with this new question, I would have preferred to have her guidance. Aengus was just four and a half, and I had no idea what had been discussed within the family.

I took a deep breath and gave the answer I felt was most age-appropriate. "Aengus, finding a heart for me was the doctor's job. I was very happy when I got the call from the doctor's office with the news that they had found a heart that seemed to be perfect for me."

There were no more questions, so I assumed that Aengus was satisfied with my answer.

I told Kristin about the conversation in case he might bring up the subject with her. Kristin then shared with me something interesting she had noticed. She said I did not use the word "my" when I referred to parts of my body. Since the transplant, she said, I referred to my heart or back or hand as "the" heart, "the" back, or "the" hand.

For instance, "My pain in the back is better now." When sharing results after an appointment, she said I made comments like "Dr. Jaski told me the heart is working very well."

I had no idea that was happening. No one else had told me I spoke differently about my body.

Kristin went on to say she'd had a long talk with a man she knew. He, also, had experienced a serious medical intervention, and had begun to feel that his body was separate from him. Fascinating!

Soon after I returned from Idaho, I headed to the San Diego airport to meet my sister. Marilyn and I spent Christmas day with my son's family. A few days later, we treated Craig's family and relatives of my daughter-in-law to dinner in downtown San Diego and a night ride in horse-drawn Cinderella carriages. In October Cousin Ed and I had seen the Cinderella carriages, their pumpkin shapes outlined with twinkling lights. We'd agreed that I just had to take my granddaughters for a ride.

With so many guests, we needed two carriages. Each of us had the special treat of riding in a carriage and seeing the beauty of the other carriage. We sang Christmas songs and waved to people walking by. The adults were in high spirits. The conversation at the restaurant was lively, and the food was delicious.

With the help of my friend Diane, who is a hypnotherapist, I later realized that I wanted to feel like a princess as much as I wanted Grace and Tori to have that unique experience.

2007, "the year of my rebirth," ended with Happy New Year hugs and good wishes for the year to come.

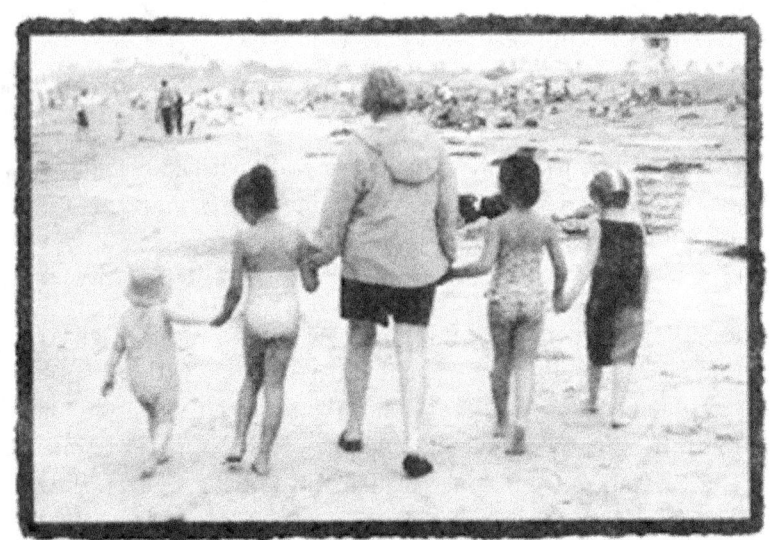

This photo was taken in 2008. The idea for the picture came to me within weeks of Petra's birth in 2006.

I had told my son about the exact photo I wanted to have of me with my grandchildren. I described the positions, with my eldest grandchild holding the hand of the youngest. My vision had us on a path among trees, walking away from the camera.

Craig said in disbelief, "Mom, you do know that Petra can't walk yet, right"? "Oh, yes. This is a picture that will be taken in a couple of years."

Craig set up the shot, but chose the beach setting that was near my home. He started to position the children. I had to correct him. Grace, looking toward Petra, made the picture even better than I had imagined two years earlier!

28
Now What?

People who have reached the point of needing an organ transplant, or faced a life threatening illness, come from all walks of life and had varying health conditions prior to the big challenge. On the other side of the surgeries and massive medicinal regimes, they each walk a unique path to recovery.

As after any trauma, mental and emotional recovery are as important and challenging as physical recovery. I'm still tightly wired, but thanks to my medical roller coaster ride I practice de-stressing activities I learned from the beautiful people I met on my journey. Throughout the three years before my transplant, and for even longer since my surgery, I have been open to trying well-being activities I've learned about in Healing Hearts, WomenHeart, my other social groups, and individual interactions.

One size does not fit all when it comes to coping skills, any more than it works for clothing. I have also found that a tip might work sometimes, but not all the time. The more tricks I put in my bag, the more options I could put into play as I stared down whatever faced me.

✶ ✶ ✶

My WomenHeart friends set up a delightful surprise for me at our regular April 2008 meeting, which happened to fall on the one-year anniversary of my heart transplant. As I walked into the restaurant I was captivated by a gigantic banner bearing the words, "For Laughing Out Loud, Linda's Heart Is Having A Birthday!"

Those words struck a special chord in me. "For crying out loud!" were the words my father bellowed when best-laid plans met an irritating obstacle. This new laughing version of that exclamation took me to the same instant happy "high" I felt whenever I gave myself the gift of laughing out loud.

The room overflowed with high-spirited women. WomenHeart members and other friends of mine had gathered more than twenty-five teddy bears and other stuffed animals for the event. After the party, Diane (my friend and surgery liaison) and I took the donations to Rady Children's Hospital, where my heart donor had been a patient.

Marilyn D. has kept our chapter alive and serves as an excellent role model. I'm grateful for the support and humor members gave me during my challenging periods. It feels good to be in the paying-it-forward phase now.

* * *

I obeyed my doctors' advice, but I also experimented with a variety of integrative health approaches as well. During small anxiety attacks in 2008, I appreciated the relief I received from a homeopathic item called Rescue Remedy. (I laughed when eight women held up their little bottles of the product at one of my support group meetings.) It helped me through several of my own traumatic events, like the day I thought I'd locked my car with the keys inside. After calling for help, I took a deep breath and a dose of RR and calmed down ... reached deeper into my purse ... and found my keys!

* * *

I faced an interesting blip in June. Out of the blue, while driving home from a health lecture, I was struck by the sudden onset of pangs of rage. Its source was a mystery to me, seemingly unrelated to anything specific in the lecture, which had addressed a wide range of recommended non-medical stress-reduction products and activities.

By the time I arrived home, I had decided to take a strong anti-anxiety pill. This was way beyond the healing scope of Rescue Remedy.

As the night wore on and sleep continued to elude me, I figured out that the dastardly culprit causing my anger was me! Why had I held on to negative remarks or situations from my past? I realized I had been a big-time grudge holder.

(In that vein, I am reminded of my mom, who gingerly tried to offer advice over the years—especially when I was in high school. She would begin with, "May I offer some constructive advice?" and I would start to cry, knowing she was about to impart some helpful guidance I truly needed.)

So why was I suddenly so angry at myself? My many notes from 2008 don't raise any specific red flags. I don't believe I was looking for people to blame for my heart condition. On the contrary, I'd been feeling grateful that my physical and emotional deterioration had contributed to my opportunity to receive a new heart, and with it a chance to become a better person.

I wrestled with my inability to stand up for myself, or for others I felt were being mistreated. Why was I such a fence sitter in arguments or debates? Why couldn't I brush off teasing or cruel remarks?

Many of the scenarios that surfaced while I remained awake that night involved trivial remarks or situations. Actually, our family had been quite tame. There was no physical or substance abuse. However, there was also very little light-heartedness, praise, or joy. I'd done my best to balance negative comments with positive encouragement.

I dumped my negative thoughts on a psychiatrist I had begun seeing in January of 2008. Frankly, I never connected with him. He sat back and said little. I detected no warmth or sign that he cared about me. (Keep in mind, I was emotionally unstable when I sought his help. He may have been an okay guy.)

There I was, releasing fury at myself for being such a wimp. When he finally managed to get in a few words, he said, "It's okay to be angry, and even depressed once in a while. You have the support and the tools you need to get better." I felt he was brushing me off.

He wasn't. He was telling me he believed in me. I don't know what else I wanted. Maybe I wanted a hug and the words, "There, there. You are a good and capable person." Actually, he did sort of say that. When a person is intent on beating herself up, love, advice, and support from others tend to fall on deaf ears until she is ready to receive help.

✶ ✶ ✶

Having avoided the gym for several months, I headed to one that had opened close to my home. I surprised my new trainer with a wild comment after my regular workout. Indulging in negative self-talk, I said, "I want to throw a tantrum!" Without any discussion, he handed me a big ball to throw as hard as I could at the wall.

Pulling tight stretch bands had me making ugly faces, sweating, and wishing I'd kept my mouth shut. He held out his hands, palms out, fingers spread upward. "Okay, see how hard you can punch my hands." he said. My arthritic punches hardly packed a wallop, especially since by this time I was roaring with laughter. Mission accomplished. A distinct high for me!

I was at home by the time I realized I was free of pain. No arthritis pain in my hands or back, and no ever-moving zinger pains below my waist. Coincidentally, I turned on the TV to the public television channel and bumped into a special about handling anger.

Still, I continued my negative self-talk well into August. Why can't I excel in anything? Why do I start projects I can't or won't finish? Why can't I focus? Why can't I sleep?

By the end of July, I was waking up each day with low back pain, reduced to nearly crawling over to take a hot shower—the only pain reliever that worked at that time. I also felt random sharp pains here and there in my body that I believed had something to do with my digestive system.

Acupuncture worked wonders for specific areas of pain. After all the needles I'd had shoved into various parts of my body, I put off trying this effective remedy until I finally succumbed to a trusted friend's encouragement to see a certified acupuncturist. The treatments brought relief from headaches and lower-back aches.

Then, after a session with the acupuncturist that failed to stop the pain below my waist, I followed his advice to go to the ER. He suspected a small gallstone, but scans showed no suspicious abdominal mass or inflammatory situation. A strong pain killer and an anti-anxiety drug were the only recommendations. I suspected flare-ups of IBS symptoms I have felt over many years.

✶ ✶ ✶

Setting out on a renewed path of pro-action, I found new activities. By August of 2008, I was participating in line dancing, a balance class, and Laughter Yoga at the senior center. Gaga and Khevin hosted a meditation session with Tibetan Singing Bowls, a beautiful and deeply calming evening. I also introduced Saturday Play Days at my home that involved a variety of non-serious games and lighthearted chatter with friends.

✶ ✶ ✶

One day I arrived for a Laughter Yoga session a little late as a result of having to comb my home several times to find my car keys. After an agitated drive to the Senior Center, I decided to take charge of my negative thoughts. Once I was settled in with the laughers, I told them I had a special request: I invited the attendees to act out having a tantrum.

I barely got out my request before, "en masse," my friends began to pound their fists, stomp their feet, and call out "No!" "Me-me-me!" and any other wails they remembered observing in two-year-olds. One fellow went down on his knees as he pounded away. They knew exactly what I'd envisioned! A lot of pent-up hostility was released in record time, followed by the most robust laughing I had heard in years!

I have since witnessed other laughter groups throwing more politically correct "tantrums." A newspaper article about the Laughter Yoga group at the Carlsbad Senior Center began with the line, "It seems that every session starts with a tantrum." Not true, but we did enjoy our authentic wailing and laughing exercise.

The foreigner in my left breast presented a new challenge: two lumps this time. I was advised to schedule a biopsy. Since 2004 I had endured a parade of mammograms, sonograms, and other tests, presumably because there was always a different person seeing or feeling my "boob cube." It would get smaller, or even dissolve, and then come back to worry the next technician or doctor.

In 2008, I stopped by Dr. Heywood's office and told him about my latest cancer scare. He was his warm and wonderful self, hugging me as he reassured me that there had been big advances in curing cancer.

Christine, a WomenHeart friend, offered to go with me to the clinic on the day of the biopsy. She decided I should go in wearing happy-face stickers. She told me to put two on my breast, right over the lurking invaders.

For extra good luck, I wore a blue and white outfit to fortify myself with Finnish *sisu* power. With purple socks on my feet and red Women-Heart scarf slung around my neck, I was ready to rumble!

Christine kept me laughing until I went in for my procedure. While my friend waited in the lobby, I sat with two nurses and a radiologist who laughed at my whimsical entrance. During the biopsy of the second lump an excited nurse announced, "It moved!"

Then I heard that the mass had crumbled. Once again, thank goodness, it was fat necrosis—nothing worse—that had brought us this scare. The nurse went out into the lobby with me to share the good report with Christine. Yea! Another high, after a scary fear-of-cancer downhill slide!

August came to a close with my rheumatologist appointment. Based on several things she saw, she told me I should not be working with hand-held weights or doing exercises that strained my hands. She recommended wrist weights, as they would be easier on my arthritic hands.

A September follow-up appointment for my painful and weak left ankle (the result of a past injury) caused my podiatrist to recommend that I stop using a treadmill and exchange my tri-level home for one with just one floor. He was surprised to learn that I was doing well wearing just a strap on my left ankle, which by now had very little cartilage. Learning that I didn't need to take daily pain pills surprised him even more. I admitted that going up or down stairs was a painful activity.

I began my search for a single-story home.

✱ ✱ ✱

"Your new heart is boring," Dr. Heywood commented in October. In his own inimitably warm style, he added, "I'm happy you got a new heart. You have such a good soul." Where was he when I was growing up and needed an encouraging daddy? His excuse would have been that he was younger than I. Picky, picky.

29
New Horizons

On January 7th, 2009, I moved into my new home. I felt good about my purchase, the beautiful grounds, the activity offerings, and the people in the community. The new wrinkle was my constant struggle to get organized. New office furniture, new bookcases, mounds of old and new paperwork—such mundane challenges reduced me to tears. I was completely undone by the everyday struggles we all face at one time or another.

My friends in the area came through with flying colors. They let me grumble, certain that I would survive. They laughed with me when I was ready to laugh at myself. Several of them got down on their hands and knees and helped me wade through papers I should have thrown out years earlier. They helped me without making me feel helpless. They treated me with compassion and dignity, making it possible for me to look back on my undignified tearful days without lasting embarrassment.

✶ ✶ ✶

Ping pong came into my life at my local senior center in 2009. Like half of those who showed up the first day, I had not played since I was a teenager. The other half were seasoned players.

Anita was the first to graciously offer coaching to anyone who wanted some help. Gradually, as we got to know each other better, some of the guys softened their competitive drive and played with us, too.

The activity was so popular that a second and then a third table had to be squeezed into the room. Eventually, the Center allowed us a second day each week.

It tickled me to hear my name called out when I entered the room. I felt like Norm walking into the bar on the "Cheers" TV series. Though my weak left ankle had to be protected and two of my falls happened in that room, I hardly ever missed a Tuesday or Friday session. Casual acquaintances felt like close friends. The desire to win was strong, but the competition never got serious enough to spoil the upbeat atmosphere as cheers, groans, and loud laughter echoed down the halls.

✳ ✳ ✳

I was becoming less critical of myself and more playful in public.

On the medical front, a whimsical spirit prevailed. I wore a spongy, red clown nose when they wheeled me to the Cath Lab in April for my second annual "big" heart check. As if that weren't enough, I also wore my purple socks and my WomenHeart red scarf. Big smiles lit up the faces of people we passed in the hospital halls. As I was being moved to the surgical table I heard, "You will have to take that off. "

"My nose?"

"No, your scarf."

✳ ✳ ✳

On the way to my sixty-ninth birthday, I had four bad falls by July. The first was in a parking lot, where I tripped over a bright yellow speed bump as I hurried to an optical (ha!) appointment. I watched the pavement moving toward my face, and did nothing to break my fall. There was a little blood, and then a nasty black eye developed that I photographed for posterity.

The second fall occurred on the brick walk near my front door. The third and fourth falls happened in a game room. For the first time, as the corner of the ping-pong table was about to gouge out my eye, I raised my left arm to shield my face.

The long string of bruises down my left side looked impressive in the photo I had a neighbor take after that fourth fall.

I went to follow-up appointments with my internist. After the last fall, I asked her whether she thought I'd had a trace of vertigo. And what did the good doctor say? "Do you feel dizzy now?"

"No."

"You are getting older. Pick up your feet," she said with a slight chuckle.

I admitted to myself that I was indeed getting older. I began walking more carefully, and, yes, "like an old woman." The good news is that as of this writing, six years later, I have not fallen again!

✳ ✳ ✳

As though time and illness had not separated us, I flew to San Francisco to reconnect with Jan and Bette, good friends from an Arizona Elderhostel session years earlier. We picked right up where we'd left off, as if we had been chatting daily. That trip included a birthday celebration for my nephew with friends and family members.

I surprised myself in July, when I enrolled in Gaga's leader-training program for Dr. Kataria's School of Laughter Yoga. Thinking I might substitute for her if she needed a break, I became a certified Laughter Yoga (LY) Leader.

By the end of the training session, visions of grandeur buzzed in my mind. I considered offering LY sessions in a senior community. I envisioned a plan to encourage church or neighborhood groups to "adopt" a community near them. Volunteers could make frequent visits, and residents and healthcare patients might feel like members of an extended family. I wanted to include laughter sessions. I came up with the name "Music, Movement, and Laughter" for group sessions.

Perhaps I would develop a nonprofit organization.

However, while I was developing self-confidence, I had none of the skills of a successful entrepreneur. In my head, my idea seemed simple. I didn't think of it as a business. I must have been off my rocker. Even nonprofit businesses have to make enough money to pay for basic supplies, media outreach, licenses, and so on.

Pushing myself into unfamiliar activities, I acquired some computer skills. I met caring people, found the help I needed to set up a website, and felt vey much alive as I reached out to dear souls who were lonely, frail, and appreciative of any attention I could provide. I set up a pilot program at a senior community and revised it many times. With the help of Donna in the healthcare center, I set up activities in different sections of the facility and was given permission to visit residents and patients in their rooms.

The staff members often reminded me that I had been volunteering for several hours. Wasn't I ready for some food or rest? There were times when I vastly overestimated my energy level, my business skills, my capacity to inspire others to volunteer with me, and my ability to make good use of the people who did try to help. Those were the times when playing ping pong was my most cathartic "health aid." I never got good at slamming the ball, but I'd double up laughing every time I tried.

✦ ✦ ✦

Toward the end of 2009 something happened that I have hesitated to share because it was so deeply personal. Yet I realize that it is the profoundly personal stories that reveal the best and the worst, that offer the most poignant insight into human experience. This story is an example of the beautiful moments people often have when they show compassion to others who have reached a low point in their lives.

Every Laughter Yoga leader in assisted living communities has stories of someone laughing for the first time in a group or of participants reaching out to help each other. The circumstances can be difficult, for many participants are in wheelchairs, hard of hearing, or in various stages of memory loss. The breakthroughs might look small to an outsider, but they are monumental to volunteers and staff who know the whole story.

Late one day I was ready to leave the healthcare section of the senior community. As I walked down the hallway, I heard a man screaming, "Get me out of here! I want to die!" I am not a trained psychologist, but I felt compelled to stop and go into his room.

I quietly walked in and asked, "May I visit with you?"

He broke off mid-yell. "Yes," he said in a near-whisper.

I don't remember how I began the conversation. I do remember that I was in his room for a long time, sitting in a chair by his bed. Almost immediately, we realized we had a lot in common. He told me about his son, who had had a heart transplant. He himself had been a "guinea pig" for stent research, while I'd had nine stents inserted before my transplant.

I noticed a cap with a WWII insignia. He told me he'd been a Marine on the Pacific front in WWII. When I shared that my father had been a SeaBee and had been there at about the same time, he praised the SeaBees' work with the Marines.

He wanted me to know that his favorite holiday was Veterans' Day, because it was the one day in the year when he felt appreciated. (Veterans' Day took on a new level of personal meaning for me as a result of that talk with him.)

There was a pause in the conversation until he asked, "Wasn't I yelling when you came in?"

"Yes," I answered.

"Didn't I say I wanted to die?"

"Yes, you did."

"Then there was the miracle."

"What did you say?" I couldn't help but ask.

He repeated all that he'd just said, ending with the miracle. Slow to realize that he was referring to me, I was dumbfounded. My memory with regard to the rest of the visit is blank. I assume I must have had tears in my eyes and given him a muttered "Thank you." I'm a good hugger, so I'm sure he got a hug and a promise that I would see him again.

I did call and talk to him a couple of times, but I was not able to see him again. Just a few days later, on my next visit, the nurse told me he had died. I said I was so sorry. Then she added that he had died a happy man because of me.

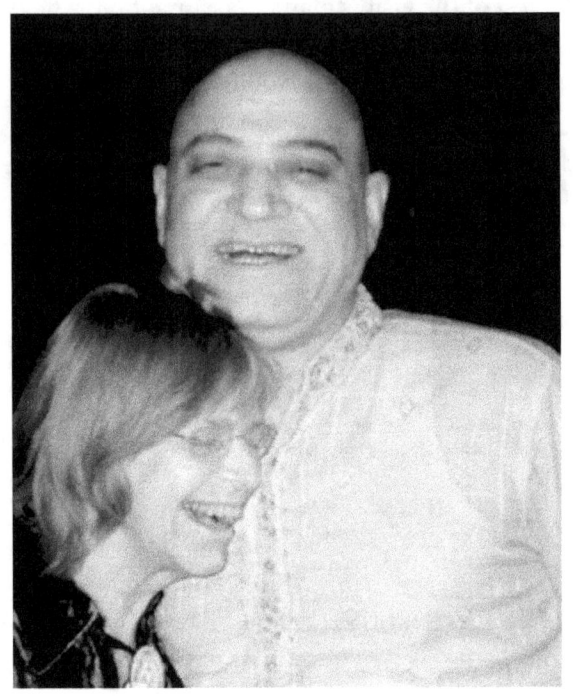

With Dr. Kataria at the Laughter Yoga Teacher
Training in Chicago

30

Moving Out of My Comfort Zone

"I'm impressed with the active life you lead," Dr. Jaski told me at my January 2010 appointment. "Especially those twice-a-week ping pong sessions of yours." I told him I was leading Laughter Yoga sessions, and he commented on my enthusiasm for the healing power of laughter. "But don't you think people might laugh too much in those sessions?" he asked. "Could people get out of control sometimes?"

"Come on, Dr. Jaski. Really?" I was amazed at his question. "You don't need to worry about that," I assured him. "The leaders have ways of bringing the craziness down if it starts to get out of hand. We end our sessions with a quiet period of deep breathing."

The more I immersed myself in Laughter Yoga, the more I realized that many people are afraid to let loose with a good belly laugh. I think they fear they might make a fool of themselves. How sad.

Most leaders have stories of people who attended a session because they knew they needed to laugh more, perhaps because they had been in families or situations where laughter was limited or nonexistent. Seeing the delight on the face of someone who's just had a good belly laugh for the first time keeps leaders on the course of spreading awareness about the physical and emotional benefits of increased laughing, even when it's done as an exercise.

* * *

One of the over-the-top highlights of my life happened in April when, with Gaga's encouragement, I signed up for a Laughter Yoga Teacher Training to be held in Chicago. The five-day program would be led by Dr. Madan Kataria, the founder of Laughter Yoga. He was coming from India to teach some leaders to move up to the level of training new leaders for local Laughter Yoga activities. I was beyond excited to have the opportunity to meet him.

I spent a glorious week with people who had experienced the "medicinal power" of laughing and understood its place in the field of integrative medicine. Dr. Kataria shared the history of Laughter Yoga and the methods he used to move groups of skeptical business people from "I'm required to attend this meeting" to lightening up and releasing work and social stress with silly laughter exercises.

The free-flowing before-breakfast laughter sessions with Dr. Kataria were magical for me. I learned I could get myself laughing even if I was alone, and that enticing myself to laugh when I was physically or emotionally upset could ease me out of a downhill slide enough to try other positive actions.

I returned to California with a new resolve to share my love and belief in laughter with people at senior and health centers who were unable to get to sessions. Back to the drawing board for me, to develop a nonprofit organization. I took business classes, joined the Chamber of Commerce, gave presentations, and set up a booth with other laughter leaders at a local city fair. Going in a gazillion directions at once, I was taxing myself with added stress. I was way out of my comfort zone.

* * *

For my 70th birthday my son and granddaughters treated me to miniature golfing, arcade games, and water-squirting boat fun at a local amusement center. The Go Karts provided the most enjoyment. Tori was with me for my first drive, but she gingerly suggested that Grace ride with me for the second round. I got the impression she was mortified by my slow speed as Craig and Grace passed us several times on the oval track.

When the starting bell sounded, Grace yelled, "Go, Grandma!" Craig and Tori passed us just once. Ha! They probably think they passed us more often, but I'm sticking to my memory of it.

* * *

Skype was just beginning to enter my life. I had done a laughter presentation at a human resources seminar. The theme that year was helping older adults become comfortable with email and the Internet and using Skype to make video calls on their cell phones, tablets, and computers.

In 2010, just seeing my grandchildren show me their pets, toys, and creative projects and tell me their favorite jokes helped me feel close to them without the hassle of making long trips or interrupting family schedules.

* * *

As I continued to celebrate the new life my new heart had made possible for me, I often got so wound up in social and business activities that I created new levels of physical and emotional stress. Exercise classes, ping pong, activities with local and distant friends, plus self-indulgent massages, manicures, and hair appointments were good for distracting me from my physical pain and vital for raising my morale.

By August, I was in serious need of emotional and physical rebalancing. Through my Chamber of Commerce activities, I learned about Dr. Anne and her "Well Being for Life" office in Carlsbad. I felt better about myself and stronger in my convictions after working with Dr. Anne. Reaching out, trying new things, and trusting in the goodness of others brought ever more beautiful people into my life.

However, even with many coping tools I ended that year with uncertainty about my chronic lower-back discomfort and ever-moving pain below the waist, which I still chalked up to my sensitive digestive system. After consulting with the Scripps Nurse Line, I gave in and went to the ER.

After a variety of scans and exams, they told me once again that there were no new problems. I was given a dose of a new-to-me pain pill, a drug used short-term to treat moderate to severe pain.

Wouldn't it be just like me to turn this ER visit into an opportunity to educate a doctor and a nurse about Laughter Yoga? Right there in the ER—my version of a safety net—I demonstrated to my captive-audience doctor how we laugh as an exercise, on purpose, because the act of laughing releases endorphins that can lessen pain.

The medical notes from that ER visit are among my favorites:

> **Hospital Records, December 4th, 2010**
>
> Again, the pain is intermittent and really only severe when she tries to change positions or get up and move. She also gives me a brochure and states she performs laugh yoga, and she continually states she is a very happy person, laughs all the time, and she would like me to do some research in the laugh yoga as she believes laughter is the best medicine … .
>
> She is resting comfortably on the gurney reading a book. During my exam, she is intermittently hypomanic with continual laughter, and at other times, very tearful and anxious appearing … .
>
> I did discuss the patient's anxiety and tearful-

> ness with the patient, but she denies any type of suicidal or homicidal ideation.
>
> She actually did sleep for one hour in the emergency department, this was the best sleep she had in a long time. I do have concerns for some hypomania[1] in this patient as she is intermittently very tearful, other times laughing uncontrollably, but she does not appear gravely disabled, and she has currently declined any psychiatric evaluation. Again, she would like me to start doing laugh yoga and has given me a brochure that I can read up on in case I would like to join her in her laugh yoga sessions.

I guess this doctor didn't realize that it was excessive pain that had caused me to burst into tears. On the other hand, my "uncontrollable laughter" was totally controlled. I was not laughing in the cubicle when I was by myself. I started to laugh when the doctor or nurse came in, just to show them that I could choose to laugh without needing a humorous prompt.

My effort to inform and interest them in the benefits of practicing Laughter Yoga had not gone well at all. Worse, my medical record now indicated a possible psychiatric instability. (At that time I was an enthusiastic new trainer of LY leaders. Eventually, I calmed down about it and did a better job of informing people properly of the physical and emotional benefits that can come from practicing Laughter Yoga.) I included the medical report because it is one of my favorite funny memories.

Oh, well. I have come to think of my craziness as an asset.

I had neglected to inform the reluctant ER doctor that in a Laughter Yoga session we balance the laughing with slow, deep, meaningful breathing. Our bodies get a thorough physical workout. I mentioned earlier that I'd left my first laughter session with Sarito feeling calm, with delightful "pop rocks," sparks of happiness, bursting inside me, lifting my mood.

The best thing about using laughter as a remedy is that it does not leave you with the negative side effects that often come with the drugs prescribed by our doctors. Not once have I ever left a laughter session and

[1] I decided to look up hypomania on webmd.com. Here's one definition: "Hypomania is a less severe form of mania. Hypomania is a mood that many don't perceive as a problem. It actually may feel pretty good. You have a greater sense of well-being and productivity. However, for someone with bipolar disorder, hypomania can evolve into mania—or can switch into serious depression."

then felt depressed. It's the other way around. When I would join a session after a bad week or while dealing with pain, I would inevitably leave feeling renewed and ready to tackle new solutions for whatever ailed me physically or emotionally. I knew I had let go and shared fun with others whose lives were as challenging as my own. Laughter Yoga is, by far, my favorite integrative medicine coping tool.

31

2011 and Beyond

Laughing, and talking about the benefits of laughing, had become part of my personal profile. Just ask Petra. During my visit to Idaho in 2011, when she was four years old, she introduced me to an adult friend of the family. "This is my grandma. She loves to laugh. It's her job."

I put off my dream of starting a nonprofit organization in February of 2011 when I was offered the opportunity to present weekly sessions of Music, Movement and Laughter at a senior community in a nearby city. I held sessions there for four years, and treasured the time I spent engaging with independent and Memory Care residents.

In April of 2011, Sarito, my first laughter "guru," introduced me to Chiwah, a fascinating writer and editor. She patiently nudged me toward writing this book. At our first meeting, she planted a seed that led me to write my first lightweight but serious little book, *7 Teasers to Get You Out of Bed*. I tossed and turned all night, pulling together a system based on the stretching and laughing exercises that energized me and made it possible for me to get out of bed in the morning with a good degree of enthusiasm. At night we make promises to accomplish projects or start habits that will improve our lives. When the morning comes, procrastination sets in. Need I say more?

✳ ✳ ✳

I began to take my Laughter Yoga spirit of fun with me wherever I went.

The time came when my ophthalmologist, Dr. Zablit, felt that my developing cataracts needed attention. Surgeries on both eyes were scheduled for May of that year (on two different days). When I learned that I would be awake during the surgeries, my fear level shot through the roof. After talking to others who had gone through cataract surgery, I calmed down a few notches.

When the eye's naturally clear lens becomes clouded, it's called a cataract. During cataract surgery, the cloudy lens is removed or cleaned out and replaced by a clear, man-made lens. It is done with local anesthesia.

When I was sitting in the pre-surgical cubicle on May 11th, I became emotional and shed some tears. The nurse asked whether I was all right. I said, "I will be." I was conscious of my history of being in "pain" from fear, and then having no problem with pain during or after a medical event.

When Dr. Zablit arrived, I asked whether I would be able to talk during the surgery. He said that would be fine.

"May I laugh?"

"Yes."

"You don't know how big I laugh."

Mission accomplished. The tension was now softened for all of us. As we were walking to the OR, I told the medical people that I worked with Laughter Yoga and explained that the goal was to get people laughing on purpose, without the need for jokes.

As I was being prepped for surgery, someone asked me what I meant about laughing without jokes. Adopting a phony professor tone, I proceeded to give a mock lecture about Dr. Madan Kataria, the doctor from India, who founded Laughter Yoga in 1995. The last thing I remember is letting out a loud "Ho-ho, ha-ha-ha."

After the surgery, back in the cubicle, the atmosphere was light. I left in high spirits. On the ride home with a friend I said, "I think I talked and laughed through the whole procedure."

My friend was with me the next day, during the post-surgery exam. In walked Dr. Zablit, wearing a big smile. "You certainly entertained us yesterday," he said. "We learned a lot about laughing." He didn't seem to be upset with me.

And what about my eye? Very good! No pain, and I was already seeing much better than before the procedure. I was actually looking forward to the surgery on my other eye, to be performed in two weeks.

The night before the second surgery, I decided I would take my camera. I had hoped to get a photo of my doctor during my post-op appointment, but there hadn't been a good opportunity. With the more relaxed atmosphere in the opthalmology department, I thought I would get the photo I wanted.

Here is where the story gets weird! Sitting in the pre-op cubicle, I took out my camera. The nurse set it on a table. Dr. Zablit noticed the camera and said, "Bring it with you." Into the OR? Really?

Just before leaving home, I'd had a way-out idea. Remember my red clown nose? In my garage I had a stash of them that our Laughter Yoga group hoped to sell at a city fair. I grabbed one, having no idea what I was going to do with it.

When they left me alone for a minute in the pre-op cubicle, I took the nose out of its package and hid it in my hand under the sheet. As we headed to the OR, the nurse got a peek at the nose and smiled.

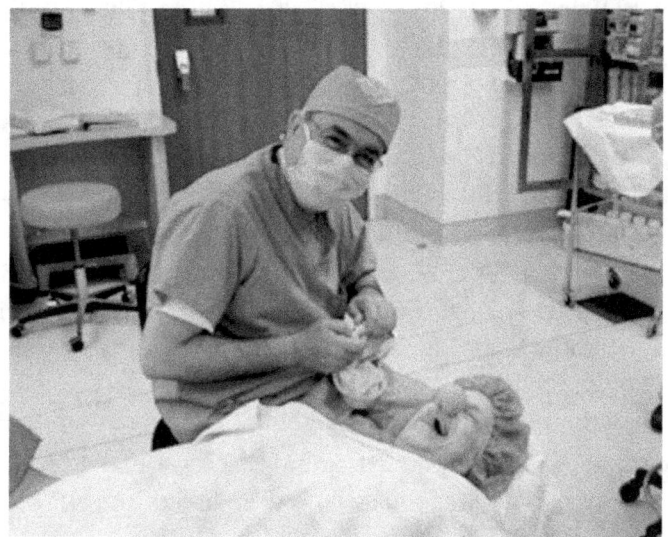

Just as before, I climbed onto the table. There was talk about what they were going to do with the camera. Someone started suggesting where each of them should stand for the photos. As my opthalmologist moved next to the table, I pulled out the nose and put it on. Everyone laughed. Funny photos were taken.

Later, I saw why the nurses had laughed while another photo was being taken. The photo showed the anesthesiologist with his hands folded, as if praying over the poor clown about to have surgery. The nurse told me he had been proposing to me! Ha!

Again, the levity lessened my tension. The camera was put away. Everyone scrubbed up, and they performed the surgery. This time I was more aware during the whole procedure. It was a fascinating experience. I talked with the doctor, but I wasn't as goofy and loud as the first time.

* * *

My intestinal system was still temperamental. An ER visit in June of 2011 ended with them giving me nothing but pain pills. Two months later, when the pains persisted, Dr. Jaski decided I should have an echocardiogram. My EF result was eighty-one percent this time! Fifty percent would be reasonable for a woman my age who hadn't undergone a heart transplant. My seventy-one-year-old body was loving my new, healthy heart!

I finally had a good talk with my GI doctor, Dr. Pressman. I told him I had read a little about the Ayurvedic holistic health system, which recommends special diets for people during periods of stress. I told him I would like to make an appointment at the Chopra Center. Dr. Pressman's response was, "It couldn't hurt."

By the time I met with Dr. Patel, a Western medicine medical doctor and an Ayurveda practitioner, on September 16th, I had read more about the system's dietary and lifestyle guidelines and had started implementing some of the suggestions. I enjoyed my talk with Dr. Patel. She confirmed what I knew and gave me additional recommendations to try.

My dietary changes carried me pain-free through a ten-minute testimonial at the 2011 All-American Laughter Yoga Conference. The theme of my talk was how laughing had helped me during my heart transplant journey. Though the hands holding my presentation notes shook like crazy, my body remained pain-free throughout the four-day conference.

I continue to have digestive issues, but I have many tools that help calm my system down. I'm good at slow, deep breathing, but I have a long way to go to be good at meditating!

* * *

Another highlight came in the form of a challenge from Dr. Heywood. He told me that a patient of his was on record for being the longest-living patient with an LVAD (left-ventricle-assist device). "I want you to be the longest-living heart transplant recipient," he said.

"Yes, sir," I agreed in a flash.

* * *

In March of 2012, having decided not to pursue setting up my own nonprofit organization, I joined the board of directors of a nonprofit organization called Laughter Matters. The founder and I had similar goals, but followed different paths of spreading awareness of laughing for emotional, social, and physical health.

I would stay on the Laughter Matters board through September of 2014, helping with presentations, substituting for laughter leaders in Laughter Matters classes, and attending workshops. I also participated in long discussions about our focus, direction, and how we might generate funding to cover the costs of providing free sessions. What an education! We were a small organization with huge dreams, facing the same growing pains that challenge most philanthropic nonprofit organizations.

✶ ✶ ✶

In 2012, Dr. Zablit told me I was in an early stage of macular degeneration. I seem to have the slow-developing form. I didn't panic, though I was not pleased to hear the news. Some of my relatives have been dealing with the same condition. My cousin Ray, who has been a great role model for staying enthusiastic about life while accepting limitations, is now in an advanced stage of macular degeneration[1] We have long, lively phone conversations.

✶ ✶ ✶

The final highlight of 2012 began with an email invitation from Donate Life to help with a new high school program to address awareness about organ donation. The staff was looking for organ recipients or their relatives to share their personal stories on the topic.

There is a dire need in our country for more people to register to be donors. The number of people who die waiting for an organ is horrifying.

Applicants for a California driver's license fill out a form that includes the opportunity to sign up to be an organ, eye, and tissue donor. Most states use a similar opt-in system, meaning that no one automatically becomes an organ donation candidate upon their death. A person has to have given legal consent. Family members may give consent after a death, but it can be a difficult decision when a loved one has just passed.

Knowing that students would be more likely to check the "yes" box on their license application if they knew the facts about organ donation, Donate Life of California had developed a presentation to be delivered by medical personnel, as well as free materials for high school teachers to present to their students.

My first meeting was held at the Life Sharing/Donate Life offices in San Diego in August. Within minutes I was captivated by what I heard from the interesting and compassionate people in the room. They told us

[1] Macular degeneration (AMD) is caused by deterioration of the retina and can severely impair vision.

about the medical personnel who conducted the high school programs and asked us to participate by speaking about our personal connection with organ donation.

As a former teacher and a heart recipient, I was eager to volunteer. My only concern was my age. Would teenagers want to listen to a seventy-two-year-old woman?

The first week of November, I received an urgent request to take part in a presentation at a high school in the San Diego area. (I think I was a last-minute substitute.)

Not having had the opportunity to observe anyone else telling a personal story, I called and emailed Donate Life staff members. My story was long, I said, with many twists and turns. What should I include? How much time would I have to deliver my message? Might I introduce humor?

The encouragement I received from staff members held me together. "You'll have between five and ten minutes, or maybe a bit longer," they told me.

I was so excited that I slept little the night before the presentation. I went in with notes for a short talk and a list of possible topics in case there was extra time. We did three sessions, with two classes present at each session. Each one opened with a well-made video of high school students, parents, and doctors discussing organ donation from many angles. Some of the students in the video shared touching personal stories.

Then came the first speaker, a trauma surgeon. Her talk included statistics about the number of people waiting for an organ transplant, information on matching donors with recipients, and other pertinent topics.

Oh my goodness, I thought, this is heavy stuff. Feeling a need to tell my personal story in a lighter tone, I opened by admitting I was nervous. I told them about the treadmill test I'd requested before I had any clue that I had heart disease. Their facial expressions told me I had their attention, and they laughed with me at some of my funny stories. That put me so much at ease that I went on for twenty minutes!

The more interest the students showed, the livelier and funnier I became. By the third session, I was almost over the top with enthusiasm. I felt that the humor I filtered in between the serious facts made it easier for them to absorb the information. They asked excellent questions.

I included an analogy about handling the emotional roller coaster ride we all travel in life. "Do not get stuck in a downhill slide. Give yourself time to be sad or angry, but get back on track as soon as possible. You have no idea how high your next high may be. Years ago, when I first put the donor's pink dot on my driver's license, I could not have imagined I would someday need a heart transplant."

I was beyond thrilled when a boy in the third session said I was his new favorite role model. He wanted to have a photo taken of us together, which we did after the presentation. A few other students got in on the photos as well.

A year later, having done many more presentations, I went back to the same high school with other volunteers. When the teacher walked over to me I said, "I think I have matured, calmed down over the last year."

"Oh, I hope not too much," he said.

Since then, I have continued to take part in high school organ donor presentations. Every session has given me such a "high"! Just ask my friends. I have no desire to be a teenager again, but meeting with them energizes me.

One of my all-time favorite compliments came during a Donate Life high school organ donation presentation.

I was getting ready to lead the third presentation of the day. The previous presenter, the mother of a teenager, who had once been a student at that same school, had survived double-lung-transplant surgery earlier in the year. She looked amazing and was an enthusiastic speaker.

During the break between classes, Bob (a heart transplant recipient) and I were handing out papers. I was fiddling with my notes. The room was large, with three classes of students settling into the long rows of folding chairs.

I made a few introductory comments and introduced Bob and myself. As I was about to start the formal presentation, I saw the raised hand of a girl far back in the room.

"Yes?"

"Are you seventy-four?"

I didn't remember saying anything about my age, but I answered, "Yes" and returned my attention to my notes.

The same hand went up again. "Are you really seventy-four years old?" Obviously, I must have made some offhand funny reference to my age as I was setting up. Once again I answered in the affirmative.

Back to my notes. I kid you not—I have witnesses! For the third time, the student said, "You are really seventy-four?" This time I became flustered and experienced a "senior moment." Had I given my correct age? In my nervousness, had I said something outrageous?

After a long pause I laughed and said, "Yes. I am really seventy-four years old, but I feel much younger, and in my head I am always laughing, singing, and dancing!"

What a great beginning to my presentations for the day!

* * *

My roller coaster ride mellowed out during 2013, the sixth year after my transplant. Was my body getting used to its new heart and the medications I required? Was I more convinced that my integrative medical coping tools worked better than going to the ER? Was I simply less fearful about my overall health? Or was I just too busy living a healthy lifestyle and interacting with upbeat people of all ages?

An event that stands out in my mind from that year was a fancy gathering for Sharp Memorial Hospital heart transplant recipients. We were honoring two men who were celebrating twenty-five years with their new hearts.

One thing I loved about this event was that it was also designed to honor the family members and caretakers whose lives had been affected by our medical journeys. For me, the highlight was having my son with me. When Craig put his arm on my shoulder while Dr. Adamson, our surgeon, was speaking, I got teary. Craig had been with me from the beginning of my rocky yet sometimes hilarious trek through the heart disease jungle.

* * *

Dr. Ehlers, who had been working with many of the Sharp Hospital heart transplant recipients, became my new primary care doctor in 2014. I had heard from several sources that he was well respected by his peers. I chose him because he had a large number of heart transplant patients. Even better, I'd learned that he had a great sense of humor.

My first opportunity to meet him came during my January appointment. His comment that tickled me the most was, "I will check only the top half of you today, since this is our first date." I soon realized that while he was witty, he was also a no-nonsense doctor. After a few sessions of hearing my rapid and enthusiastic speaking style, he told me to try meditating to loosen my tightly coiled body and mind.

He made it clear that organ recipients have to be ever vigilant about changes in our health. The sooner anomalies are detected, the sooner they can be dealt with, resulting in a better chance of survival. Feeling well is good; we just have to be careful not to let down our guard.

The anti-rejection medicines make organ recipients sitting ducks for all forms of cancer. Skin cancer is most likely to find us. Regular dermatology checkups are mandatory. My scare in 2013 involved almost missing basal cell carcinoma on my scalp and over my right eye. Casual comments during exams brought a second look from my doctor. Basal cell carcinomas are the easiest to treat, but they do need to be caught as soon as possible. Had the doctor not noticed the spot over my eye, it could have gone undetected for a year.

I feel relatively safe under the care of my new dermatologist, Dr. Mona Mofid, who is also Medical Director of the American Melanoma foundation. Her medical expertise and refreshing personality fit me well.

I had already begun wearing a medical alert necklace at home. Since I lived alone, I'd decided to get a necklace with a "help" button I could push if I fell or needed help making a medical decision.

Next came "Help" devices that can be used outside the home. People are surprised to learn about my GPS connecting device. I like knowing I can be in touch quickly with someone who can keep me calm and help me connect with a family member, doctor, or ambulance. The safety net of a push-one-button system makes me feel comfortable driving to evening events and going places at a distance from my home.

I had stopped going to the gym when my rheumatologist and my podiatrist both warned me that I needed to protect my hands, my lower back, and my weak ankle. Learning about a locally owned gym near my home awakened in me a desire to work with a trainer again. I signed up the next day. Left to my own devices, I do not move enough during the week.

The atmosphere in the smaller, more personal gym was perfect for me. I have learned that exercising is tolerable (okay, fun) if I am allowed to talk a mile a minute to young, good-looking male trainers. They have been able to push me, and even make me sweat sometimes, as long as I can laugh at myself and at the earnest trainers. I look forward to my early-morning workouts in the gym and the interactions with others who work out alongside me.

With each passing year stiffness increases after sitting a long time or getting some sleep. The instinct is to remain still and not aggravate your knees, ankles, or back. I try to visualize a phrase I once heard: motion is lotion. Even small movements have a lubricating effect. I've read that the secret to vital aging is to keep moving.

I think I was not a fan of disco music when it was introduced. Now, at age seventy-five with "appropriate behavior" filters removed, I have discovered a delightful morning elixir. My TV is set to the Retro Disco music channel. My alarm goes off, and the TV or CD player is turned on.

Okay. I may wince when the spirited music invades my ears. My fingers start tapping, I begin to turn from side to side. As more parts of my body join the fun, I can't help but smile. I laugh at myself and start to sing. Soon I am sitting up, making bigger movements with my arms and legs. When I add the laughing, the energizing supply of fresh oxygen gives me a noticeable energy boost, setting me up for a good day.

The guys at the gym will testify that I usually arrive at 7:30 in the morning with a big smile on my face and a bounce in my step.

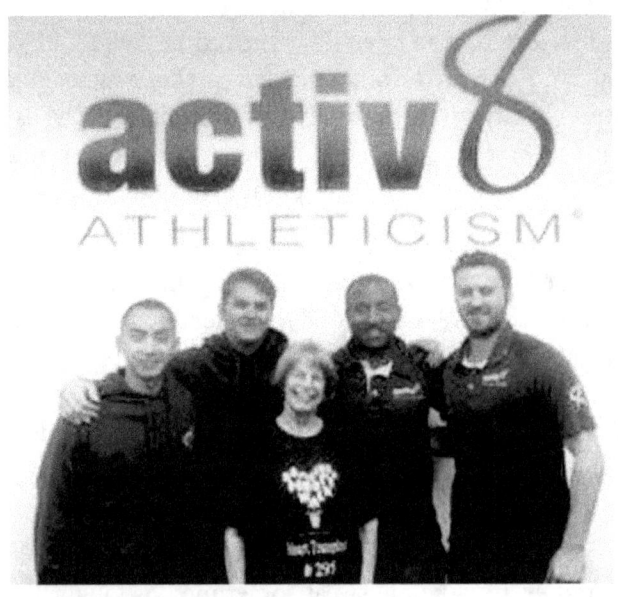

32

From Surviving to Thriving

After being offered the possibility of a heart transplant at the age of sixty-six, I'd been told that my cardiologists had predicted in late 2006 that I had two to three years left to live with my weakening heart. I didn't panic. I quickly decided I wanted to learn more and start the transplant evaluation process.

I have received the gift of living past my expiration date. I am seventy-five, and still alive! Along with benefiting from good health, I have developed a variety of life skills that have taken me to a happy and productive state. For the first time, I can honestly say I like and approve of myself.

Well, maybe not every minute of every day ... .

Do I still get in trouble at times for saying or doing the wrong thing? Yes, but now I listen, think about how I can use the information, correct my action if possible, and move on. I don't beat myself up the way I did in the past.

Just as I was about to tackle this section of the writing, I almost tripped over an unexpected gift from the universe. I had been reading the June 1, 2015, issue of *TIME* magazine and left it open on the floor to the next section, oblivious to the images and words on the exposed pages.

Now I saw that the left-hand page showed a deflated red balloon, and under it the word "BOUNCE." On the right-hand page floated an inflated balloon (patched with a cross made of two bandage strips) floating over the word "BACK." In smaller letters at the bottom of the left-hand page was the sentence, "Scientists now know why some people rebound so well from setbacks." A corresponding sentence on the right-hand page read, "They also know how the rest of us can be more like them."

Hmmm!

I snatched up the magazine and devoured the five-page article by Mandy Oaklander.

The first three pages described who I had been most of my life, who I have become, and how I got to where I am today.

My pat phrase had been, "I have been hampered in reaching my goals because I've always had low self-esteem, lacked self-confidence." Yet I had trouble believing that. I knew I was good enough in the areas of intelligence, talent, and appearance. I had not come from a family that continually put me down. I'd never never been abused. I wasn't competitive, but I did envy people who appeared to be self-assured.

After reading the article, I realized that it was not self-esteem I lacked. According to Dr. Dennis Charney, co-author of "Resilience: the Science of Mastering Life's Greatest Challenges," what I'd lacked was "resilience," a set of skills that make it possible for people to not only get through hard times but to thrive during and after them.

Dr. Steven Southwick, the co-author, had written, "The vast majority of us will be faced with one or more major traumatic stressors during a lifetime. But the countless smaller stresses also take a toll."

The article told of scientific studies in which scans showed significant brain changes during and after stressful situations. The brains of participants who received resilience training were able to change for the better.

In the revision of their book, the authors emphasized that having a strong social network was *critical* to developing resilience, whereas in the past it had been considered "nice but unnecessary."

How was this relevant to me? During my medical journey I had progressed from having a few San Diego acquaintances to receiving help from a large social circle. Friends surrounded me with physical and emotional support and then accepted my help when I was ready to be there for them.

The researchers had found that people could develop resilience skills that would fortify them during stressful times. The article offered tips for doing that.

Two skill sets emphasized in the article were regular exercise and mindfulness.

How did this apply to me? Walking, strength training, and playing ping pong had increased my activity level far beyond what it had been in earlier years.

Mindfulness has been described as the practice of purposely focusing attention on the present moment and accepting it without judgment.

What this meant to me: On my medical journey I became aware of mindfulness, breathing awareness, and meditation when I was looking for ways to decrease my tightly coiled, nervous demeanor. When I sense that I am becoming overwhelmed, I try slow, deep breathing while silently repeating a calming phrase. I plan to look deeper into mindfulness training.

✳ ✳ ✳

To make it easier to see why I felt the *TIME* article was so relevant to me, I will compare the ten "Expert Tips for Resilience" from the article with examples of actions I took during my heart transplant roller coaster ride:

1. **"Develop a core set of beliefs that nothing can shake, developing an ethical code to guide daily decisions."**

   • Long before my heart problem emerged, I had believed that the gift of life obligated me to do whatever I could, in big or small ways, to make the world a better place. Acting on my desire to help others as I had been helped brought me immense pleasure. I accepted a variety of volunteering experiences, enjoying time spent with people both older and much younger than I was.

   • Looking back at isolated happenings during my recovery involving the interaction of gifted and caring people and help from a higher power strengthened a core belief that I am a small piece in a huge, interconnected picture. I hurt for people who feel it necessary to fight to defend their differences rather than come together to acknowledge their similarities.

2. **"Try to find meaning in whatever stressful or traumatic thing has happened."**

   • I think my desire to write this book fits this tip. On hearing my funny, informative, and inspirational stories, my friends had told me that my attitude and recollections might help others to see new ways to handle the stresses in their lives.

3. **"Try to maintain a positive outlook."**

   • Decades ago, when my mother and I were watching Willard Scott honoring people celebrating their 100th or older birthdays on *The Today Show*, my mom commented that she didn't want to live that long. Without hesitation, I said, "I do!"

   • Dr. Heywood said I had "The Gratitude Attitude."

• Dr. Kataria's Laughter Yoga tips encouraged us to start the morning laughing. I took seriously his advice to spread to others the joy that laughter brought us.

• I wrote *7 Teasers to Get You Out of Bed* to introduce people to stretching, laughing, and singing first thing in the morning to boost their energy and mood.

4. "Take cues from someone who is especially resilient."

• The first person who came to my mind when I read this was my mother. It was she who held the family together after the death of her young son and, later, after the death of her husband. She handled her challenges with strength and without complaint.

• After our father died, my sister Marilyn, then sixteen, weathered, if not happily, leaving her friends when we moved to California. Our finances were iffy just when she was hoping to go to college. To save money, she worked, went to a community college, and sewed her own clothes until she could afford to earn her bachelor's and master's degrees at the colleges of her choice. Meanwhile, she (though I didn't realize it at the time) was the one who gave me social tips and encouragement. She taught me to drive well enough to earn my license on my first try. My mother was teaching, and VA benefits were available to help me attend Occidental College without having to get a job. I had it easier. My self-confidence and strength under fire were not tested. Over the years, I have told my sister how proud of her I have always been.

5. "Don't run from things that scare you. Face them."

• When in the middle of an emotional situation I made worse each time I tried to find a solution, I turned to "Ozzie's Words of Wisdom." (Ozzie was our support group leader in the Scripps Integrative Medicine Healing Hearts Program.) "Much of the stress in our lives," he said, "is because we choose problems we cannot solve rather than accept solutions we do not like." With respect to some tangles, knowing I was as much at fault as the other parties, I finally chose to back away from situations and people I had hoped to appease.

• Asking whether I could talk and laugh during my first cataract surgery helped me conquer my fear. Later, I wore a red clown nose in the OR just minutes before my second cataract surgery began.

• I said "Yes!" to heart transplant surgery even though I had experienced complications during and after bypass surgery.

6. **"Be quick to reach out for support when things go haywire."**

• I joined Healing Hearts, WomenHeart, and Heart Transplant support groups.

• Close friends came to my aid when I became overwhelmed while trying to organize paperwork in my new home. I have learned to set aside my pride and ask for help.

7. **"Learn new things."**

• I took training to be a Laughter Yoga leader.

• From Dr. Madan Kataria, founder of Laughter Yoga, I took the next-level training that qualified me to teach future leaders.

• I developed and led Music, Movement, and Laughter sessions at three senior communities.

• I took training to give high school organ donation presentations sponsored by Donate Life of California.

• I was elected to the board of directors of two nonprofit organizations: Laughter Matters and the Pulmonary Transplant Foundation.

• With neighbors, I learned how to play hand bells so we could offer local holiday music concerts.

• I learned how to ride/drive a Segway in order to go on a tour in Las Vegas.

8. **"Find an exercise regimen you'll stick to."**

• I walk in the morning with neighbors.

• I do strength training at a gym, following my strict rule of working only with young male trainers who let me talk and laugh during my workouts!

• To make sure I get frequent bursts of movement, I do stretching and dancing while in bed or sitting on a chair, always with bouncy music.

9. **"Don't beat yourself up or dwell on the past."**

• I'm getting better at accepting responsibility without taking all the blame for relationships that don't work out.

• I am realizing I don't have to take on views that don't fit my values.

• I'm improving at releasing emotional stress.

10. "Recognize what makes you uniquely strong—and own it."

- I'm high on life. I recognize possibilities more often than I run from obstacles.

- I've been told I am a mood raiser in most situations.

- I enjoy close friendships within a wide age range,
resulting in a variety of conversation and and activities.

My enthusiasm seems over the top at times. I try to reel myself in, but I get caught up in the moment. I am a one-women percussion set. When my activities are over I head home to wind down, flopping on my bed at any time of day or night. I need a break from me!

When I finally gave up hoping everyone would like me, I began to find people I could relate to, people traveling paths similar to my own. Now that I am no longer looking for them, I see loving, caring, and funny people everywhere I go. Were people like that always within my reach?

Thank goodness, years ago I did find a few people who could put up with me and my insecurities. They have witnessed my changes and growth. Better yet, they have remained my close friends.

Was it divine intervention that caused me to put off completing the writing of my book for so long? Toward the end of writing and editing, in the middle of my week-long seventy-fifth birthday treat from my daughter, I realized I had to wait until we could spend more time together. We chose to meet in Las Vegas, where we saw amazing shows, ate tasty treats, and had unique adventures while we talked, laughed, and walked with few breaks.

Our daily obligations were forgotten. Kristin seemed to enjoy being with the open and carefree person I had become. She took photos of me having fun with performers, servers, and other tourists. We returned to our respective homes, sharing stories with friends about how much playfulness we'd seen in each other.

In April 2016 I was seventy-five years old and celebrated nine amazing years with a heart transplant. It was time to have my thorough annual checkup, with catheters examining both sides of my heart.

A photo was taken while I was waiting for my neighbor to arrive and take me home. It was late afternoon. The atmosphere was light, and I began to tell stories and share photos that showed how grateful I was to have had this medical miracle experience. The next thing I knew, my adorable female nurse set up the photo opportunity. I do enjoy being with young men!

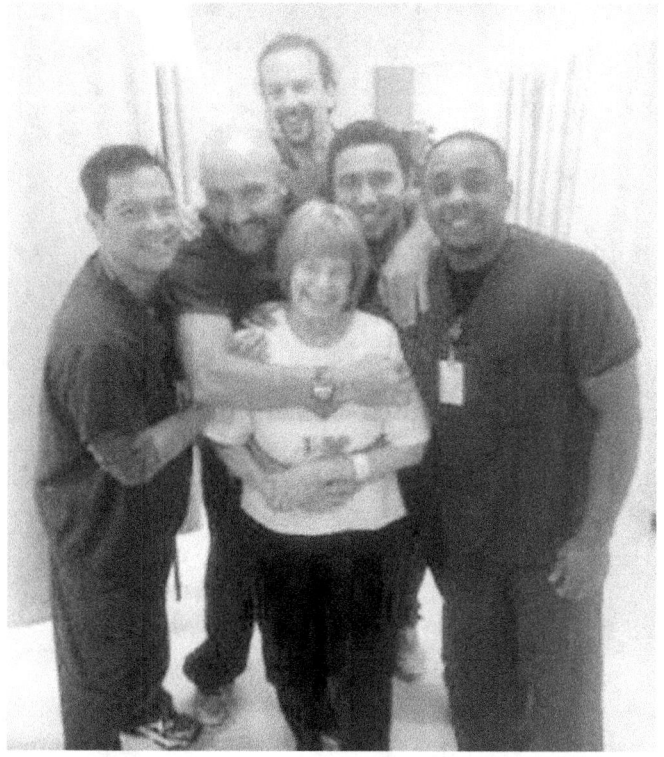

Thanks to the resilience I have been developing and the beautiful people who have entered my life, I truly believe that I have gone beyond surviving ... to thriving!

33

My Sincere Plea

If you have not yet registered to be an organ donor, please be aware of the urgent need for a huge donor pool. Lives are lost while people wait for a lifesaving organ. Encourage others to understand the need, get the facts, and register to be a donor.

Registering online is the fastest and easiest way to make your wishes known. Go online to: www.organdonor.gov.

Facts to Ponder:

In your lifetime, you are far more likely to need an eye, tissue, or organ donation than to be a match for a recipient.

When you are admitted to a hospital, the number one priority is to save your life, not to harvest your organs.

Organs are allocated according to medical need, blood and tissue type, and height and weight. Celebrity status and wealth are not considered.

One person can save eight lives and enhance the lives of fifty others through organ, eye, and tissue donation.

Organ transplants are lifesaving operations. People on the transplant waiting list are suffering organ failure from conditions such as heart failure and kidney disease. Without the help of a generous gift of life from an organ donor, they will die.

Tissue transplants are lifesaving and/or life-enhancing operations. They save the lives of recovering burn victims, help blind people to see, and allow people to walk again.

Post-transplant organ, eye, and tissue recipients can live healthy, active lives that weren't possible when they were ill. Most recipients make such an amazing recovery, you would not know that they received a transplant unless they told you.

Anyone can become a potential organ donor regardless of age, ethnicity, or medical history.

All major religions support or permit organ, eye, and tissue donation.

There is no discrimination due to sex, occupation, or social or financial status when determining who receives an organ.

There is no cost to the donor or their family.

For the more than 123,000 Americans currently waiting for an organ, an organ transplant is their only remaining medical option. On average, 150 people are added to the nation's organ transplant waiting list each day—that's one every ten minutes. Sadly, an average of twenty-two patients die every day while waiting, simply because the organ they needed was not donated in time.

Approximately eighty-one organ transplants take place every day in the United States. That's more than 29,000 people who begin new lives a year! A living donor can provide a kidney or a portion of their liver, lung, pancreas, or intestine to someone in need.

More than one-third of all deceased donors are age fifty or older, and nearly ten percent are age sixty-five or older. More than one million tissue transplants are performed each year, and the surgical need for tissue has been steadily rising. Corneal transplants, meanwhile, restore sight to 50,000 people each year.

* * *

Participating in high school presentations is rewarding, fun, and a meaningful way for me express my appreciation to my heart donor and her family.

Before I talk, the students have listened to serious information. Interaction starts with their questions and comments. We try to have a speaker who can share a personal story about being or knowing a recipient or a donor. The subject becomes real before their eyes. Humor sneaks in, especially as I finish my testimonial.

I ask the students whether it is still "cool" to recycle. Being polite to the "old" lady, they give me the thumbs-up sign. I bring out my dark green shirt, saying, "Look what I won during a Donate Life activity."

Then I ask for a drum roll as I show the back of the shirt, which bears a large recycle-triangle symbol with a gingerbread-like figure in the center.

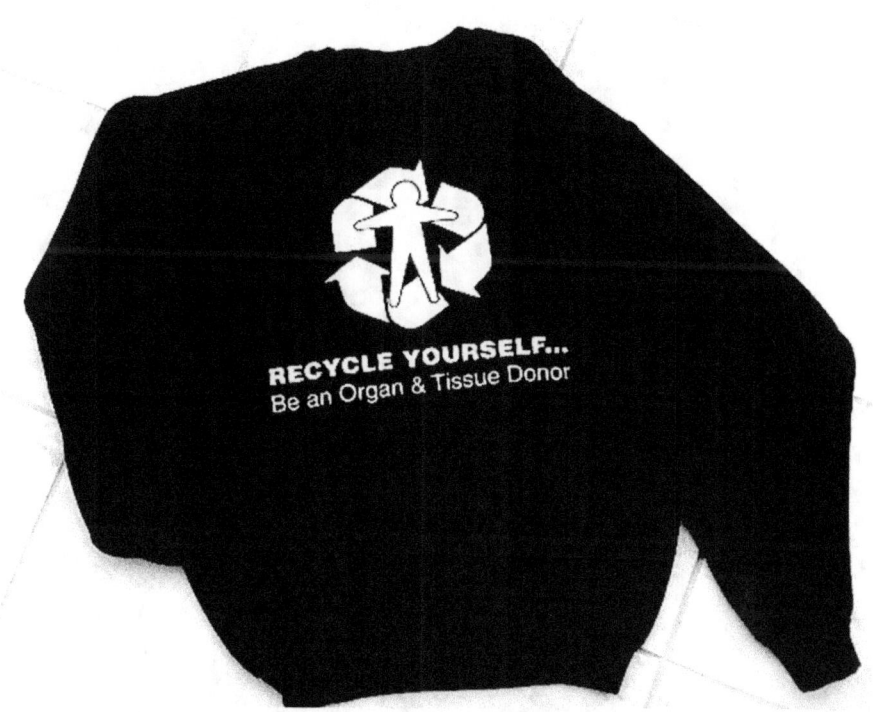

Cheers and laughter erupt. I frequently get hugs from students as they leave the room. By the time I return to my car, I'm feeling "higher than a kite!"

So ... let me ask YOU: Are you a recycler? If so, go online now to www. organdonor.gov and register to recycle yourself. Use the search box to go to the page for your state.

THE END

A Word from the Author

If you would like to share a reaction to one of my stories, I would enjoy hearing from you. Did you try something I'd done to raise my spirits? What have you done that I might want to try? Tell me about:

- a doctor or nurse who was extra special

- a personal funny story

- a crazy spirit raiser that works for you

- a sweet reaction of a child to your condition

- a spiritual experience you would like to share

- tricks you use to move often while lying down or sitting

- a personal donor or recipient experience involving an organ, tissue or eye transplant

I will not share what you write to me unless you give me permission.

If I sense a growing interest in sharing and supporting each other in our medical and aging challenges, I may start an interaction, invitation-only Laughing Hearts Facebook Group. We can use videos to offer a sense of community that might be especially important for people who aren't able to get out with friends as often as they did in the past.

LaughingHearts4us@icloud.com